CONTROVERSIES in CANCER

Design of Trials and Treatment

CONTROVERSIES
in
CANCER

Design of Trials
and Treatment

Edited by

Henri J. Tagnon, M.D.

Maurice J. Staquet, M.D.

Masson Publishing USA, Inc.

New York • Paris • Barcelona • Milan • Mexico City • Rio de Janeiro

Proceedings of an EORTC Symposium held in Brussels,
Belgium, April 26–29, 1978

ISBN 0-89352-049-7

Library of Congress Catalog Card Number: 79-84480

Printed in the United States of America

Acknowledgment

The EORTC Foundation will receive all royalties
from sales of this book.
The authors freely gave their time
and received no remuneration.
We are extremely grateful to all of them.

M. J. Staquet
European Organization for
Research on Treatment of Cancer,
Brussels, Belgium

Contributors

S. J. ARNOTT
Western General Hospital
Crewe Road
Edinburgh EH4 2XU
Great Britain

K. BREUR
Wilhelmina Gasthuis
Eerste Helmersstraat 104
Amsterdam-Oud-West
The Netherlands

G. BRITTINGER
Hämatologische Abteilung
Medizinische Universitätsklinik Essen
Hufelandstrasse 55
4300 Essen 1
Western Germany

R. BURKHARDT
Gemeinnütziges Gemeinschaftskrankenhaus
Herdecke
Beckweg 4
5804 Herdecke
Western Germany

D. P. BYAR
Head, Clinical and Diagnostic Trials Section
Biometry Branch
National Cancer Institute, NIH
Landow Building, Room C-509
Bethesda, Maryland 20014
U.S.A.

G. P. CANELLOS
Chief of Medicine
Sidney Farber Cancer Institute
Harvard Medical School
44 Binney Street
Boston, Massachusetts 02115
U.S.A.

S. E. COME
Division of Medical Oncology
Sidney Farber Cancer Institute
Harvard Medical School
44 Binney Street
Boston, Massachusetts 02115
U.S.A.

W. GAUS
Universität Ulm
Klinische Dokumentation
Prittwitzstrasse 6
7900 Ulm/Donau
Western Germany

A. GOLDIN
Division of Cancer Treatment
National Cancer Institute
Bethesda, Maryland 20014
U.S.A.

D. GONZALEZ
Wilhelmina Gasthuis
Eerste Helmersstraat 104
Amsterdam-Oud-West
The Netherlands

A. M. GUARINO
Division of Cancer Treatment
National Cancer Institute
Bethesda, Maryland 20014
U.S.A.

G. A. HIGGINS
Veterans Administration Hospital
50 Irving St. N.W.
Washington, D.C. 20422
U.S.A.

C. HILL
Institut Gustave Roussy
16bis, av. Paul-Vaillant-Couturier
94800 Villejuif
France

D. R. JONES
Institute of Cancer Research
Division of Epidemiology
Clifton Avenue
Sutton, Surrey
Great Britain

KIEL LYMPHOMA GROUP
c/o Division of Haematology
Department of Medicine
Universität Essen
Hufelandstrasse 55
4300 Essen 1
Western Germany

G. KIENLE
Gemeinnütziges Gemeinschaftskrankenhaus
Herdecke
Beckweg 4
5804 Herdecke
Western Germany

J. KLASTERSKY
Institut Jules Bordet
1 rue Héger-Bordet
1000 Bruxelles
Belgium

F. J. LEJEUNE
Institut Jules Bordet
1 rue Héger-Bordet
1000 Bruxelles
Belgium

D. MACHIN
EORTC Data Center
Institut Jules Bordet
1 rue Héger-Bordet
1000 Bruxelles
Belgium

F. MARTIN
Laboratoire d'Immunologie et
de Médecine Expérimentale
Faculté de Médecine
7 boulevard Jeanne d'Arc
21033 Dijon
France

L. NORTON
Department of Neoplastic Diseases
Mount Sinai School of Medicine
New York, N.Y.
U.S.A.

M. PALMER
Christie Hospital and
Holt Radium Institute
Withington
Manchester M20 9BX
Great Britain

S. J. POCOCK
Department of Clinical Epidemiology
and Social Medicine
The Royal Free Hospital
21 Pond Street
London NW3 2PN
Great Britain

R. J. PRESCOTT
Medical Computing and
Statistics Unit
Medical School
Teviot Place
Edinburgh EH8 9AG
Great Britain

M. ROZENCWEIG
Division of Cancer Treatment
National Cancer Institute
Bethesda, Maryland 20014
U.S.A.

H. SANCHO-GARNIER
Institut Gustave Roussy
16 bis, av-Paul Vaillant-Couturier
94800 Villejuif
France

P. SCHEIN
Division of Medical Oncology
Vincent T. Lombardi
Cancer Research Center
Georgetown University
School of Medicine
Washington, D.C. 20007
U.S.A.

R. SIMON
Division of Cancer Treatment
National Cancer Institute
Bethesda, Maryland 20014
U.S.A.

M. J. STAQUET
EORTC Data Center
Institut Jules Bordet
1 rue Héger-Bordet
1000 Bruxelles
Belgium

A. M. STARK
Department of Gynaecological
Oncology
Queen Elisabeth Hospital
Gateshead, Tyne and Wear
Great Britain

M. W. STEARNS, Jr.
Chief, Rectum and Colon Service
Memorial Sloan-Kettering Cancer
Center
New York, N.Y.
U.S.A.

R. J. SYLVESTER
EORTC Data Center
Institut Jules Bordet
1 rue Héger-Bordet
1000 Bruxelles
Belgium

E. van der SCHUEREN
Wilhelmina Gasthuis
Eerste Helmersstraat 104
Amsterdam-Oud-West
The Netherlands

L. M. van PUTTEN
Radiobiological Institute TNO
Lange Kleiweg 151
Rijswijk (ZH)
The Netherlands

U. VERONESI
Istituto Nazionale dei Tumori
via Venezian 1
20133 Milano
Italy

J. WHITEHEAD
Department of Mathematics
Chelsea College
University of London
Manresa Road
London SW3
Great Britain

Contents

1

Applications of Large-Sample Sequential Tests To The Analysis Of Survival Data

D. R. Jones

Institute of Cancer Research
Division of Epidemiology
Sutton, Surrey, England

J. Whitehead

Department of Mathematics
Chelsea College
University of London England

INTRODUCTION

IN THIS PAPER WE PRESENT a sequential version of the logrank test; that is, a sequential procedure for the comparison of two sets of survival data, under the assumption of proportional hazards. In developing this theory we have found a general class of large-sample sequential tests, which includes a version of the modified Wilcoxon test of Gehan[4,5] as another special case.

The derivation of the general method was motivated by Robbins'[10] treatment of the comparison of two Bernoulli populations. It is based on an analogy with the case of normal random variables with mean θ and variance 1.

SEQUENTIAL TESTS FOR A NORMAL MEAN

Consider a sequence $x_1, x_2, \ldots,$ of normal random variables with mean θ and variance 1. The hypotheses $H_0:\theta < 0$ and $H_1:\theta > 0$ can be tested sequentially in the following symmetric manner (see Fig. 1). Put $S_n = x_1 + \cdots + x_n$, and plot S_n against n. If S_n ever exceeds some constant value a, stop the test and accept H_1. If S_n ever falls below $-a$, stop and accept H_0. This test will stop with probability one.

The operating characteristic, $c(\theta) = P_\theta(H_0$ is accepted), can be found as follows:

$$c(\theta) = \sum_{n=1}^{\infty} P_{\theta}(H_0 \text{ is accepted}, N = n)$$

$$= \sum_{n=1}^{\infty} \int_{\mathcal{A}_n} f_n(\mathbf{x}_n; \theta)d\mathbf{x}_n \tag{1}$$

where

N = terminal sample size,

$\mathcal{A}_n$ = space of samples $\mathbf{x}_n \equiv (x_1, \ldots, x_n)$ for which H_0 is accepted with $N = n$, and $f_n(\mathbf{x}_n; \theta)$ = joint density of $\mathbf{x}_n$.

Now, for normal random variables with mean θ and variance 1

$$f_n(\mathbf{x}_n; \theta) \propto \exp(\theta S_n - \tfrac{1}{2}\theta^2 n) \tag{2}$$

so that

$$\frac{f_n(\mathbf{x}_n; \theta)}{f_n(\mathbf{x}_n; -\theta)} = \exp(2\theta S_n)$$

On $\mathcal{A}_n$, *ignoring overshoot*, $S_n \doteq -a$. Thus, from (1),

$$c(\theta) \doteq \sum_{n=1}^{\infty} \int_{\mathcal{A}_n} e^{-2\theta a} f_n(\mathbf{x}_n; -\theta)d\mathbf{x}_n$$

$$= e^{-2\theta a} c(-\theta)$$

By the symmetry of the test, $c(-\theta) = 1 - c(\theta)$, and so

$$c(\theta) \doteq 1/(e^{2\theta a} + 1), \quad \text{for all } \theta \tag{3}$$

Note that expression (3) has been derived using only the form of the joint density, or the likelihood function, given in (2) together with the assumption of no overshoot. Using a little more structure, and invoking Wald's lemma, the following expression for average sample number can be derived,

$$E_{\theta}N \doteq \begin{cases} \dfrac{a(e^{2\theta a} - 1)}{\theta(e^{2\theta a} + 1)}, & \theta \neq 0 \\[2ex] a^2, & \theta = 0 \end{cases} \tag{4}$$

Tests on the normal mean can be performed by plotting S_n against n and using any of the boundaries shown in Figures 1–4. Expressions for the operating characteristic can be found for any of these, using only the form of $f_n(\mathbf{x}_n; \theta)$ given by (2), and the assumption of no overshoot. Skew triangular regions, and combinations thereof for three hypothesis tests can also be evaluated in this way.

In choosing stopping regions, the properties required for the test can be formulated as specifications on the value of $c(\theta)$ at two points. Among tests satisfying these specifications the test of Figure 2 will be optimal in the sense that it minimizes $E_{\theta}N$ at both these fixed points.[3] The test of Figure 4, or a skew version of it, will be optimal in the sense that it asymptotically (as $a \to \infty$) minimizes max $E_{\theta}N$, which occurs at some value of θ between

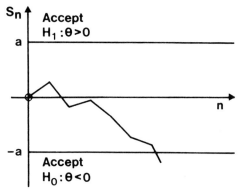

FIG. 1

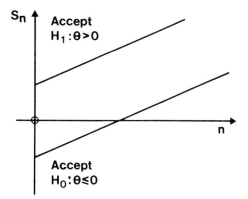

FIG. 2. Wald's sequential probability ratio test.[13]

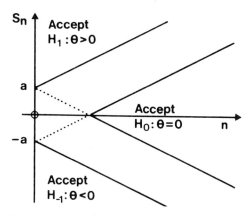

FIG. 3. Sobel and Wald's test of three hypotheses.[12]

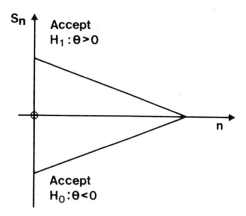

FIG. 4. Anderson's modified sequential probability ratio test.[1] See also Lawing and David.[8]

the fixed points.[7] It is because of these optimality results, and the ease of finding approximate, but adequate, operating characteristic and average sample number functions that these regions are suggested.

THE SEQUENTIAL LOGRANK TEST

In general, let $x_1, x_2, \ldots,$ be any sequence of observations, and suppose that the joint density $f_n(x_n; \theta)$ of the first n of them is parameterized by the real parameter θ. Let

$$l_n(\theta) = \log f_n(x_n; \theta) \tag{5}$$

Then, if θ is small,

$$l_n(\theta) = \text{const} + \theta Z - \tfrac{1}{2}\theta^2 V + O(\theta^3)$$

where

$$Z = \frac{dl_n}{d\theta}\Big|_{\theta=0} \tag{6}$$

and

$$V = -\frac{d^2 l_n}{d\theta^2}\Big|_{\theta=0} \tag{7}$$

Thus

$$f_n(x_n; \theta) \propto [\exp(\theta Z - \tfrac{1}{2}\theta^2 V)][1 + O(\theta^3)] \tag{8}$$

For small θ, $f_n(x_n; \theta)$ has the same form as the normal likelihood (2), with Z replacing S_n and V replacing n. This suggests the use of sequential plans based on plotting Z against V using any of the boundaries in Figures 1–4. The derivations of operating characteristics will be valid up to overshoot and up to terms in θ^3. The average sample number functions for the normal case will give a guide to the expected terminal value of V.

The general method is a sequential analogue of Rao's large-sample, fixed-sample like-lihood-ratio test[9] and is reported in Whitehead.[14]

In the logrank case we assume that there are two sets of survival data, both subject to the same conditions of censoring and represented by survivor functions $\mathcal{F}(t; \theta)$ and $\mathcal{F}(t; -\theta)$ where

$$\mathcal{F}(t; \theta) = [\mathcal{H}(t)]^{1-\theta/2} \qquad (t > 0)$$

and $\mathcal{H}(t)$ is a survivor function on $(0, \infty)$.

Expressions (6) and (7) yield

$$Z = -n_1 + \sum_{i=1}^{k} A_{i1} = n_2 - \sum_{i=1}^{k} A_{i2}$$

and

$$V = \sum_{i=1}^{k} A_{i1} A_{i2}$$

where there are, at the time of plotting Z and V, k deaths after survival times of $t_1 < \cdots < t_k$; n_j being in set j, and A_{ij} is the proportion of patients *known* to have survived a time $\geq t_i$ that belongs to set j ($j = 1, 2$). Thus Z and V are the fixed-sample logrank statistic and its variance, as presented by Cox, Section 7.[2]

This test, and a sequential modified Wilcoxon test, are discussed at greater length in Ref. 6, which also includes results of simulations performed to assess the accuracy of expressions (3) and (4) for trials of realistic dimensions. The simulated tests involved plotting Z against V on a diagram similar to Figure 1. Patients entered the trial according to a Poisson process, parameter 50, and were assigned to treatment at random. The treatment groups were given exponential survival times, parameters $1 - \frac{1}{2}\theta$ and $1 + \frac{1}{2}\theta$. Each trial was simulated 200 times. When $\theta = 0$, the situation corresponds roughly to a trial with a mean survival time of one year and patients entering at a rate of one per week.

The values $a = 6$ and $\theta = 0, 0.1$, and 0.5 were among those simulated, and for these (3) gives $c(\theta) = 0.5, 0.231$, and 0.002, respectively. Using the estimation method suggested by Siegmund,[11] the data yielded the estimates $\hat{c}(\theta) = 0.525, 0.206$, and 0.002, respectively, from the 200 replications. Investigations using a simpler patient entry procedure and larger numbers of replications indicate closer agreement and are described in Ref. 6. The predictions of the theory would appear to be adequate for practical purposes.

It can also be shown that, if the number of deaths in set j at termination is n_j^* and the terminal value of V is V^*, then

$$E_\theta n_1^* \doteq \frac{2E_\theta V^*}{1 + \frac{1}{2}\theta} \quad \text{and} \quad E_\theta n_2^* \doteq \frac{2E_\theta V^*}{1 - \frac{1}{2}\theta} \tag{9}$$

Using (4) to give $E_\theta V^*$, and then (9), the theory predicts that for the three θ values $E_\theta n_1^* = 72.0, 67.8$, and 31.7 and $E_\theta n_2^* = 72.0, 61.3$, and 19.0. These are to be compared with simulated mean values for n_1^* of $76.5, 68.9$, and 30.9 and for n_2^* of $75.7, 66.8$, and 22.1. The predictions give a rough guide to the mean numbers of deaths sufficiently accurate to be of considerable use in the planning of a sequential trial.

REFERENCES

1. Anderson, T.W. (1960). A modification of the sequential probability ratio test to reduce sample size. *Ann Math Statist*, **31**: 165–97.

2. Cox, D.R. (1972). Regression models and life-tables. *J Roy Statist Soc*, B **34**: 187–202.

3. Ferguson, T.S. (1967). *Mathematical Statistics: A Decision Theoretic Approach*, Academic Press, New York.

4. Gehan, E.A. (1965a). A generalised Wilcoxon test for comparing arbitrarily singly-censored samples. *Biometrika*, **52**: 203–23.

5. Gehan, E.A. (1965b). A generalised two-sample Wilcoxon test for doubly-censored data. *Biometrika*, **52**: 650–53.

6. Jones, D.R., and Whitehead, J. (1979). Sequential forms of the logrank and modified Wilcoxon tests for censored data. *Biometrika*, **66** (in press).

7. Lai, T.L. (1973). Optimal stopping and sequential tests which minimize the maximum expected sample size. *Ann Statist*, **1**: 659–73.

8. Lawing, W.D., and David, H.T. (1966). Likelihood-ratio computations of operating characteristics. *Ann Math Statist*, **37**: 1704–16.

9. Rao, C.R. (1947). Large-sample tests of statistical hypotheses concerning several parameters with application to the problem of estimation. *Proc Camb Phil Soc*, **44**: 50–57.

10. Robbins, H. (1974). A sequential test for two binomial proportions. *Proc Natl Acad Sci USA*, **7**: 4435–36.

11. Siegmund, D. (1976). Importance sampling in the Monte Carlo study of sequential tests. *Ann Statist*, **4**: 673–84.

12. Sobel, M., and Wald, A. (1949). A sequential decision procedure for choosing one of three hypotheses concerning the unknown mean of a normal distribution. *Ann Math Statist*, **20**: 502–22.

13. Wald, A. (1947). *Sequential Analysis*, John Wiley, New York.

14. Whitehead, J. (1978). Large-sample sequential methods with application to the analysis of 2 × 2 contingency tables. *Biometrika*, **65**: 351–6.

2

Advantages And Defects of Single-Center And Multicenter Clinical Trials

D. Machin, M. J. Staquet, and R. J. Sylvester

EORTC Data Center
Institut Jules Bordet
1 Rue Heger—Bordet
Bruxelles 1000, Belgium

INTRODUCTION

ALTHOUGH THE EORTC ITSELF has been in existence since 1962, it wasn't until January, 1974, that the EORTC Data Center began operation. In the beginning the staff consisted of a director, a statistician, and a secretary. Today the staff of 14 comprises a director, two statisticians, two computer analysts, four full-time and three part-time data managers, and two secretaries.

One of the principal functions of the EORTC (although by no means the only one) is to encourage developments in the treatment of cancer by means of multicenter, multinational, randomized clinical trials. The EORTC Data Center was set up specifically to service such trials. This work includes the design and review of new clinical trials, the design of data forms, patient randomization; data collection, management, and storage; preparation of administrative and interim statistical reports; the preparation of a final statistical report, and help in preparing a final published report. At this time the Data Center is monitoring approximately 60 multicenter clinical trials with data on over 5,000 patients and has a further 10 protocols in advanced stages of planning. Thus the Data Center itself has a strong incentive to support the multicenter clinical trial.

The object of this paper is to review the advantages and disadvantages of single-center and multicenter clinical trials from the clinical, management, and statistical points of view. Some of the clinical and management aspects have been briefly reviewed elsewhere by Staquet[5] and practical problems have been discussed by George.[3]

CLINICAL ASPECTS

The Advantages of a Single-Center Trial

It is obviously a great advantage, if one is preparing a new protocol, to have all the physicians who are to be involved in its operation located in the same institute. Consultation with everyone involved is then easy, and it should be possible to obtain quick agreement on the final form of the protocol. The protocol can also be written to suit the particular center in such a way as to make maximal use of the facilities available. Only institutional review is necessary, and no international agreement on the ethics involved is required.

Once the protocol is approved there need be no delay in making it operational, and once operational, it is relatively easy to monitor the protocol so that all the criteria are adhered to and all eligible patients from that institute are entered. If necessary, ambiguities can be clarified and modifications to the protocol can be quickly made as the trial progresses.

Another advantage is that the attending physicians may be in a position to see all the patients entering on a trial. Also, they can easily review all the patient material and any missing data can be obtained without difficulty. Toxicities can be readily monitored.

The trial can be quickly closed to patient entry. If, for example, unexpected and unacceptable toxicities become apparent or if substantial treatment differences occur and it would be unethical to continue with the inferior treatment.

Disadvantages of a Single-Center Trial

In the design stage the protocol may not benefit from the experiences of others with the proposed treatments, or of comments that an external review body may give.

If the center is small, recruitment for a trial may be very slow or indeed may be insufficient to mount a trial at all, and certainly not one with more than two arms.

Some essential medical facilities may be lacking and adequate statistical, computer and data management services may not exist.

It may be difficult to convince others of the validity of the trial conclusions or to extend the results to the wider patient population, perhaps leading to a repeat of the trial by other single centers or in a multicenter trial.

Advantages of a Multicenter Clinical Trial

When a protocol is prepared for a multicenter trial, it is discussed by many experienced clinicians from many centers, and these experiences will be reflected in the final version of the protocol. The protocol is then reviewed (within the EORTC at least) by external assessors who may themselves contribute to the design of the final protocol. Discussion of the proposed protocol can often lead to beneficial changes in some procedures within a particular institute and to standardization of others (perhaps a common classification of pathology).

Often certain specialized facilities or treatments (e.g., BCG) are available in only a few centers but can be made available to other centers through the cooperative group.

Multicenter trials enable small centers to contribute to the trials; they also allow the possibility of randomized trials in rare tumors.

Multicenter trials will have, in general, a greater accrual rate of patients than a corresponding unicenter trial. This allows the possibility of very large trials of relatively short duration and trials with more than two arms.

Multicenter trials can be completed in a shorter period of time, thus minimizing the possibility of change with time of the characteristics of the patients in the study.

The sooner a trial can be completed the less the chance that participants will lose interest in the trial.

A multicenter trial allows the comparison of results from one center with another and eventually affords the possibility of generalizing these results to a wider patient population. Differences in results between centers may lead to closer examination of the data, which may reveal additional information on both the disease process and its treatment.

Cooperative trials lead to more cooperation and exchange of information among participating centers, as well as to discussion of current practice and care within the different centers. Such discussions can improve both the standards of the trial and the general standards of patient treatment.

In multicenter trials there is often a review of all patient records by the trial coordinator or a small committee established for this purpose. There may also be a central pathology review.

Because of the relatively speedy accrual rate onto a trial, unexpected toxicities can be quickly evaluated and placed in the context of all patients undergoing the particular treatment regimen. If a participating clinician finds unacceptable toxicity in the first patients entered on trial he may decide the treatment must be stopped, whereas if the clinician learns that no other centers have this particular problem, he or she may feel it to be more a function of the particular patients treated than of the treatment itself.

Multicenter discussions may prevent unnecessary duplication of effort by reducing the possibility that several centers will independently carry out essentially the same trial.

Central statistical, computer, and data management facilities may be available which could not be provided on a comparable scale even in large single centers.

Once the results of a trial are established, there is immediate use of these results by the members of the cooperative group and a wider acceptability of the results by the medical community at large.

Disadvantages of Multicenter Clinical Trials

Multicenter trials are difficult to organize; it takes a long time to reach agreement on a final protocol, and, once agreed upon, it may take a long time to become operational.

Protocol design is usually a complicated undertaking. Most investigators participating in a cooperative trial have their own ideas on selection of patients and alternative treatment modalities.

In a cooperative group, the presence of people from different disciplines and different backgrounds (e.g., surgeons, radiotherapists, chemotherapists) can leave the definition of the aims of the study either too imprecise or too ambitious. This can lead to protocols with too many stratifications, too many alternative treatments, and the imposition of complex rules which cannot then be implemented.

It is difficult, in the multicenter approach, to check that all patients are receiving treatment as specified in the protocol, and any missing data are often difficult to retreive. There may be differences from one center to another in the evaluation of the results with respect to therapeutic response and toxicity.

Meetings of trial participants are expensive and time consuming.

In multinational trials there are usually long distances between investigating centers. Language differences may also add to the difficulties and costs of multicenter trials. There may be also different "ethical" codes, which must either be reconciled or lead to the exclusion of a particular country from a particular protocol.

STATISTICAL ASPECTS

Estimating Between Center Variability by Analysis of Variance

For ease of presentation we will assume that we are discussing a multicenter trial with two arms and that the response variable is a normal random variable, following Chakravorti and Grizzle:[2]

$$y_{ijk} = \mu + t_i + b_j + c_{ij} + e_{ijk} \tag{1}$$

where $i = 1, 2; j = 1, 2, \ldots, m; k = 1, 2, \ldots, n_{ij}; y_{ijk}$ is the observation on patient k from institute j on treatment i; μ is the overall effect; t_i is the fixed effect of the ith treatment; b_j is the effect of the jth institute, assumed to be random and distributed as $N(0, \sigma_b^2)$; c_{ij} is the interaction effect of the ith treatment and jth institute, assumed to be random and distributed as $N(0, \omega^2)$ and e_{ijk} is the random error component distributed as $N(0, \sigma^2)$. All components are assumed to be independently distributed. The object of the clinical trial is to test the hypothesis $H_0: t_1 = t_2$ against the alternative $H_1: t_1 \neq t_2$. Chakravorti and Grizzle[2] discuss how the variance components may be estimated in general. If $n_{ij} = n$ for all i and j, they reduce to the analysis of variance estimates given by Kempthorne,[4] which are summarized in Table I.

It is clear from Table I that if we wish to test for differences between the treatments, that is, differences between treatments *averaged over all possible institutes*, we would use the criteria T/I, which has an F distribution with 1 and $m - 1$ degrees of freedom.

The best estimate of $t_1 - t_2$ is given by the corresponding difference of observed treatment

TABLE I
Structure of Analysis of Variance[a]

Source of variation	Degrees of freedom	Mean square	Expectation of mean square
Institutes	$m - 1$	H	$\sigma^2 + 2n\sigma_b^2$
Treatments	1	T	$\sigma^2 + n\omega^2 + \frac{1}{2} nm (t_1 - t_2)^2$
Treatments × Institutes	$m - 1$	I	$\sigma^2 + n\omega^2$
Error	$2m(n - 1)$	E	σ^2
Total	$2mn - 1$		

[a] For a clinical trial involving several centers (equal number of patients/center).

means $\bar{y}_{1..} - \bar{y}_{2..}$, and which has a variance

$$V = 2\left(\frac{\omega^2}{m} + \frac{\sigma^2}{mn}\right) \tag{2}$$

It should be noted that if ω^2 is large relative to σ^2 then to minimize V it is advisable to include a large number of institutes in the trial.

In actual practice the participating institutes are not selected as a random sample of all possible institutes, so that the test for differences between treatments for the *institutes that have participated* is T/E, which has an F distribution with 1 and $2m(n-1)$ degrees of freedom. The estimate of the treatment comparison remains $\bar{y}_{1..} - \bar{y}_{2..}$, but now the variance for the particular participating institutes is $2\sigma^2/mn$.

The variance attached to an estimate therefore depends on the use to which the estimate will be put.

If we wish to predict the "gain" an individual patient can expect by receiving treatment 1 rather than treatment 2, then this is given (with the corresponding standard error) by

$$(\bar{y}_{1..} - \bar{y}_{2..}) \pm \left\{2\left[\frac{\hat{\sigma}^2}{mn} + \hat{\omega}^2\left(1 + \frac{1}{m}\right)\right]\right\}^{1/2} \tag{3}$$

Thus, to estimate this gain we need to estimate ω^2 and hence implicitly make the assumption that indeed the participating institutes *are* a random sample.

How Many Centers?

Suppose we have m centers in a two-arm multicenter trial in which each center contributes $2n$ patients (n per arm). The total entry per arm, $N = mn$, is fixed and we design the trial in such a way that

$$V = 2\left(\frac{\omega^2}{m} + \frac{\sigma^2}{mn}\right)$$

is minimized simultaneously with the cost C, which we assume is of the form

$$C = \alpha'm + 2\beta'mn + 2\gamma'n \tag{4}$$

where α' is the fixed cost per participating center, β' is the cost per patient treated, and γ' is the cost related to the duration of the trial. In actual practice β' may turn out to be the smallest cost.

We will assume it takes twice as long to enter two patients as one for a particular institute.

We minimize, therefore,

$$VC = 2\left(\frac{\omega^2}{m} + \frac{\sigma^2}{mn}\right)(\alpha'm + 2\beta'mn + 2\gamma'n) \tag{5}$$

or, writing $\phi = \omega^2/\sigma^2$, $\beta = 2\beta'/\alpha'$, $\gamma = 2\gamma'/\alpha'$, $N = mn$, and $P = VC/2\alpha'\sigma^2$,

$$P = \left(\frac{\phi}{m} + \frac{1}{N}\right)\left(m + \beta N + \gamma\frac{N}{m}\right) \tag{6}$$

with respect to m. Differentiating P and setting the resulting expression to zero gives

TABLE II
Variation in "Optimal" Number of Participating Centers for $N = 100$, $\phi = 1$

β	γ	Number of centers m	Number of patients per arm per center n	P
1	1	101.5	1.0^-	4.0
0.5	1	73.3	1.4	2.9
0	1	28.4	3.5	1.4
0.5	0.75	72.7	1.4	2.9
0.25	0.75	53.4	1.9	2.8
0	0.75	25.7	3.9	1.4
0.25	0.5	52.1	1.9	2.3
0.125	0.5	39.4	2.5	1.9
0	0.5	22.3	4.5	1.3
0.125	0.25	37.5	2.7	1.9
0.0625	0.25	28.7	3.5	1.6
0	0.25	17.6	5.7	1.3
0.05	0.1	24.3	4.1	1.5
0.025	0.1	19.1	5.2	1.4
0	0.1	12.9	7.8	1.2

TABLE III
Variation of P [a]

Number of centers m	Number of patients per arm per center n	P
1	100	11.11
2	50	3.57
4	25	1.69
5	20	1.47
10	10	1.21
20	5	1.23
25	4	1.27
50	2	1.51
100	1	2.00

[a] With possible designs for $N = 100$, $\phi = 1$, $\beta = 0$, $\gamma = 0.1$.

$$m^3 - N(\phi\beta N + \gamma)m - 2\phi\gamma N^2 = 0 \tag{7}$$

which can be solved for m, the number of centers, for given N, ϕ, β, and γ.

Table II summarizes some solutions to this equation for $N = 100$, $\phi = 1$, together with the corresponding P. It is clear that the "optimal" number of centers increases as both β and γ increase.

For $\beta = 0$, $\gamma = 0.1$ the optimal design is $m = 12.9$, $n = 7.8$; with $P = 1.197$. The "costs" of the nearest practical designs are for $m = 12$, $n = 8$, $N = 96$, $P = 1.200$, and for $m = 13$, $n = 8$, $N = 104$, $P = 1.194$.

Of more interest than Table II perhaps is the variation in P for different m and n with fixed $N = mn$ and fixed relative costs β and γ.

Table III shows the variation in P for the possible designs with $N = 100$, $\phi = 1$ and $\beta = 0$, $\gamma = 0.1$.

The optimum is $m = n = 10$, but P differs little from its minimum of 1.21 when either $m = 20$ or $m = 25$. The highest relative value of $P = 11.11$ is the unicenter trial $m = 1$, $n = 100$.

The Influence of Unknown Prognostic Factors

Again we assume that $2n$ patients from each of m ($\geqslant 1$) centers are randomly allocated to two treatments in equal proportions within each center. We also assume that the response y to treatment depends not only on the treatment given but also on the value of some prognostic variable x by means of the following linear model:

$$y_{ijk} = \alpha_i + \beta_i x_{ijk} + \epsilon_{ijk} \tag{8}$$

where $i = 1.2$; $j = 1, 2, \ldots, m$; $k = 1, 2, \ldots, n$.

The α_i, β_i are the treatment effects and regression coefficients, respectively, and ϵ_{ijk} is the random error component distributed as $N(0, \sigma^2)$.

This model assumes that any institute effect expresses itself as a prognostic factor through the corresponding x_{ijk} for a particular patient given a particular treatment by a particular institute.

Now if the prognostic variable x_{ijk} is not measured (perhaps its value was not appreciated at the beginning of the trial, or it is some entirely unknown variable, which therefore could not have been measured), then its influence cannot be assessed using Equation (8).

If however we assume such prognostic variables are *not* present, i.e., $\beta_1 = \beta_2 = 0$, the hypothesis of the equality of α_1 and α_2 (i.e., no treatment differences) can be tested by assuming

$$u = (\bar{y}_{1..} - \bar{y}_{2..})/(2\sigma^2/mn)^{1/2} \tag{9}$$

is $N(0, 1)$ random variable.

We here assume σ^2 is known. However, if we were to estimate it, that estimate would be inflated by the presence of any influencing prognostic variable not accounted for in the model, since then $(\beta_i x_{ijk} + \epsilon_{ijk})$ would be taken as the random element in Equation (8).

Now, if β_1, β_2 are not zero, then the expected value of the random variable corresponding to u is

$$E\{u\} = \frac{(\alpha_1 - \alpha_2) + (\beta_1 \bar{x}_{1..} - \beta_2 \bar{x}_{2..})}{(2\sigma^2/mn)^{1/2}}$$

which, under the null hypothesis of no treatment differences, becomes

$$B = \frac{(\beta_1 \bar{x}_{1..} - \beta_2 \bar{x}_{2..})}{(2\sigma^2/mn)^{1/2}} \tag{10}$$

If the prognostic variables are influential but are not measured, then the bias B will be unknown and, if large, may lead to false conclusions concerning the relative efficacy of the treatments by use of Equation (9).

If the prognostic variables themselves are random variables (see Atiquillah[1]) and

$$x_{ijk} = \mu_j + \eta_{ijk} \tag{11}$$

where μ_j is an institute mean for the prognostic factor and $E\{\mu_j\} = \mu$, $\text{var}\{\mu_j\} = \sigma_\mu^2$, and $E\{\eta_{ijk}\} = 0$, $\text{var}\{\eta_{ijk}\} = \sigma_\eta^2$, then the expected value of the bias *is*

$$E\{B\} = \frac{(\beta_1 - \beta_2)\mu}{(2\sigma/mn)^{1/2}} \tag{12}$$

The variance of the bias is

$$\text{var}\{B\} = \left(\frac{\beta_1^2 + \beta_2^2}{2\sigma^2}\right)(n\sigma_\mu^2 + \sigma_\eta^2) \tag{13}$$

which does not depend on the number of institutes, but only on the number of patients per institute.

For the particular case $\beta_1 = \beta_2 = \beta$, although the expectation of the bias is now zero, the variance is not; its value is proportional to β^2.

For fixed $N = mn$ then, Equation (13) has its maximum when $m = 1$, $n = 100$, that is, a unicenter trial, and its minimum when $m = 100$ and $n = 1$. The reason for this is clear. If a prognostic variable can range over the interval $[a, b]$, say, for the population at large, but only over a subinterval of this interval within a particular institute, then patients entering on trial, who are from that institute only, cannot reflect so well the patient population at large. It is therefore important that, if the institute of treatment does have prognostic significance, an institution effect must be included in the model; by implication multicenter participation in the trial is required.

Statistical Disadvantages of Multicenter Trials

The statistical arguments we have presented, although by no means complete, suggest that multicenter trials are more desirable than unicenter trials, but the cost argument depends critically on the entry rate cost, and the prognostic argument depends on an uneven distribution of prognostic variables between centers.

Some statistical disadvantages of multicenter trials are

1. subsequent analysis and possibly interpretation of the results are more difficult;
2. possible extra unaccounted-for variability, which will inflate error (e.g., wide differences in entry rate from center to center);

3. it is more difficult to use sequential designs and adaptive treatment assignments;
4. the use of "historical controls" is less likely.

CONCLUSION

In summary, the clinical arguments in favor of multicenter trials far outweigh those for unicenter trials. This does not imply that in appropriate circumstances unicenter trials should not be performed but rather that multicenter trials should be the norm for Phase III trials of the type usually performed in cancer patients.

The statistical arguments for multicenter trials hinge on the need for large trials and the generalization of the results of such trials to the wider patient population.

What is important is that both the physicians and statisticians working in the area of multicenter clinical trials know *both* the advantages and disadvantages of such trials, and those who conduct only unicenter trials should be made aware of their limitations.

REFERENCES

1. Atiquillah, M. (1964). The robustness of the covariance analysis of a one-way classification. *Biometrika*, **51**: 365–72.

2. Chakravorti, S.R., and Grizzle, J.E. (1975). Analysis of data from multiclinic experiments. *Biometrics*, **31**: 325–38.

3. George, S.L. (1976). Practical problems in the design, conduct and analysis of cooperative clinical trials *Proc. 9th nt. Biometric Conf.*, **1**: 227–44.

4. Kempthorne, O. (1965). *The Design and Analysis of Experiments*, Wiley, New York.

5. Staquet, M. (1976). The practice of cooperative clinical trials. *Europ J Cancer*, **12**: 241–43.

3

The Experience of the EORTC-Gnotobiotic Project Group in Planning, Organizing, Performing, and Evaluating Cooperative Clinical Trials

Wilhelm Gaus

Universität Ulm Klinische Dokumentation
Ulm/Donau, Western Germany

A. INTRODUCTION

1. Motto and Thesis

Most beginners in biostatistics think that the statistical test is most important in the evaluation of a trial. Later on the design of the study is felt to be most essential. For cooperative clinical studies we think the organization and monitoring is most critical.

2. The Problems of Cooperative Trials

The problems in cooperative and multicenter trials are in principle the same problems as in single-center studies, but they are more difficult to handle and control. It is especially more difficult

1. to get samples of the same statistical population of patients in all participating hospitals
2. to observe the same points and use the same laboratory methods in all participating hospitals
3. to ensure the same treatment, the same standard of nursing care, and the same environmental conditions in all participating hospitals
4. to get a small "variance within treatments" due to the differences among hospitals, their organization and structure, the language barrier, and the different attitudes of the patients
5. to combine democratic methods with a straightforward procedure

17

B. COUNTERMEASURES

1. Detailed Protocol

The protocol of a cooperative study must be much more detailed than that of a single-center study. Although the Gnotobiotic Project Group has some experience, it needs one to two years to develop a new protocol. The protocol must be accepted unanimously by the representatives so that the Study Coordinator or the statistician can apply the protocol strictly. The protocol is published at the beginning of the study not only to tell colleagues that a study on this specific topic is on the way, but to enable everybody to check what was originally planned, what was actually done later on, and which hypotheses were indeed independent of the data.

2. Minimum Requirements

The protocol should not demand procedures that are too difficult; otherwise the clinical units are overcharged and are not able to fulfill the requirements. The protocol, finally, contains only the "minimal requirements" that are thought necessary to answer the matter in question. But all participating hospitals should be able and willing to fulfill the few minimal requirements correctly.

3. Minimum Number of Cases

A specific task of the protocol is to set up a minimum number of complete cases per unit. The cases of those hospitals that are unable to contribute this minimum number are not evaluated because the statistical power of the trial is decreased more by the variance added by those units than it is increased by a few more cases. Additionally we feel that hospitals with only a few cases have not enough experience in delivering gnotobiotic care. In contrast to some other papers of this symposium we feel that it is not best to incorporate as many units as possible, because the main goal is not to estimate the variance between units but to estimate the treatment effect.

4. Central Randomization

The Statistical Center does a central randomization. It is done via telephone or telex. Both the Statistical Center and the clinical unit fill out the admission form to document the randomization. The central randomization enables a better stratification, and all withdrawals from the trial are known. Consequently, the Statistical Center knows at any time how the study is going on, quickly recognizing when a unit becomes less active, and can handle requests for late records.

5. Forms

According to the regulations of the protocol, a set of forms is developed for each study. The forms are a part of the protocol and have several functions:

1. They grasp and document the relevant data and function as "interface" between the clinical units and the data processing.
2. They are a checklist for the clinical physician and bring the regulations of the protocol back to his attention.

3. The completed forms allow the Statistical Center to monitor whether or not the clinical units are following the protocol.

A set of forms consists of different types of forms, which have to be filled out at certain times or at different intervals during the period when the patient is being investigated. The structure of a patient's record is usually:

1. admission (for eligibility, stratification, randomization)
2. first day (for detailed information on the patient and his disease)
3. daily, weekly reports, etc. (for control of the treatment and the course of the development of the disease)
4. follow-up and/or termination of the treatment (for the determination of the therapeutic success)
5. forms for special purposes (service centers)

The admission form is also available from patients who are not willing to participate in the study as well as from all withdrawals, all rejected patients, drop-outs, early deaths, etc.

All forms have a column for coding and for keypunching. In the Statistical Center, the Medical Data Administrator of the study transfers the information obtained from the clinical personnel to this column. One reason for the manual coding is that according to our experience the forms must be checked very carefully by a Medical Data Administrator before computer input. After coding, the original form is submitted to keypunching. The idea is to do all the steps on the same piece of paper, starting with the obtaining of data from the patient through keypunching. This saves efforts in data-transfer, data-labeling, and data-linking and minimizes the errors introduced by these steps. We prefer manual coding because mark-sensing or OCR forms are not flexible enough and/or not always handled correctly in the wards.

6. Data Checking

Immediately after the last form is filled out, the record is sent to the Statistical Center. If necessary, the Statistical Center reminds the unit representative of the record. The records are checked in the Statistical Center for completeness, correct sequence of the forms, plausibility, and accordance with the protocol, immediately after receiving them. Questions are cleared with the clinical units. Then nonnumerical data are coded, and all data are keypunched. After input of the data to a computerized source file via a data editor program, the data are checked again.

These steps have to be pursued continuously during the course of the study, beginning as soon as a randomized case is accepted and the complete patient record is received. This method allows the course of the trial to be carefully monitored.

7. Service Centers

The service centers perform special tasks which are either totally unavailable or not available in a adequately standardized way in the individual clinical units. Service centers might be: statistical center, pharmacy, quality control board, chemical laboratories, bacteriological laboratories, etc.

8. On-Study Group

For each clinical unit a representative is nominated. The representatives are responsible for ensuring that their individual unit adheres to the protocol on the one hand and maintains the interest of their unit in the study on the other hand. The representatives of the clinical units and of the service centers form the *On-Study Group*. The chairman of the On-Study Group is the Study Coordinator. The On-Study Group meets twice a year. At the meetings the Statistical Center reports on the state of the study but not on preliminary results. The On-Study Group is the highest authority of the study. Changes and extensions of the protocol—if indeed unavoidable—are decided by the group unanimously. Between meetings the Study Coordinator is responsible for monitoring the study and making operational decisions if necessary.

9. Data Processing and EDP-File Organization

The procedure for loading the data on the computer must be flexible because the data come more or less continously throughout the study. To permit this flexibility the data are first stored in a computerized *source file*, which is structured exactly like the patient's own records. Each block of the source file starts with the patient's number, the type of the form, and the appropriate calendar date.

When a patient's record is added to the source file, it is always treated by a program for the formal checking of the data. This program is universal; it can check single records or complete source files. The conditions of checking are stored in a parameter file. Thus the program can be used for different studies by using different parameter files.

Conditions of checking for each variable can be

1. range
2. illegal values within the range
3. legal values out of the range

Conditions for checking for any pair of variables can be

1. illegal combination (e.g., male and pregnancy)
2. necessary combination (e.g., if the variable "fever?" is answered with "yes," then the variable "temperature" may not be blank)
3. definition of more than one range for the same variable. The range actually used depends on another variable.

For any variable, any number of conditions of checking may be used. Thus detailed conditions can be installed.

For the evaluation, a binary random access file is produced from the source file. It may contain more blocks than the source file. These extra blocks are necessary because some forms have to be split up into several blocks in order to get block sizes that are not too different. The EDP job creating the random access file generates additionally an address table. Two function-subroutines use the address table (a) for the computation of the block address and (b) for the determination of how many forms of a certain type are available from a certain patient. Thus the blocks of the random access file are accessed by block number from the view of the operating system, but from the view of the user programs they are accessed by patient number, type of the form, and a running number starting from 1 for each patient × type-of-form combination. Programs are developed for generating contingency tables and some other data-descriptive procedures by dialog or parameter cards. Finally, subsets of data can be transferred to standard files in order to use them with programs from statistical packages (e.g., BMD or SPSS).

10. Hypotheses Testing

Because of the randomization procedure the Statistical Center also has a completed admission form of the rejected and omitted patients. A statistical analysis of the content of these forms is performed in order to check whether or not the on-study and evaluated cases may be considered as an unbiased sample of all eligible patients.

If it is impossible to standardize all components of the treatment (e.g., up to the present time the cytostatic treatment of acute leukemia has been constantly under investigation; treatment changes frequently, and there is no generally accepted scheme), these not standardized components are recorded in full detail. Therefore we have the possibility of controlling statistically and retrospectively whether or not the groups are comparable in those components of the treatment that are not *a priori* standardized. For this purpose of controlling the comparability of groups we do tests which are not orthogonal.

For the *a priori* chosen variables which measure the treatment success, the suitable statistical procedures for hypothesis testing have to be applied. In case the test is not significant, the likelihood functions should be computed. Then a definite statement can be made as to which maximal treatment effect has been overlooked.

11. Data Snooping

Besides the classical testing of hypotheses, we do some "data snooping" to generate new hypotheses. For this purpose quite often several hundred tables are produced and sometimes even more. For this reason appropriate programs for frequency distribution and its parameters, for contingency tables, or for fitting curves to time-dependent data are available. Of course, in reporting the results a careful distinction must be made between *a priori* hypotheses proved by the study and hypotheses generated by the study.

C. CONCLUSIONS

1. Permanent Statistician

Cooperative multiclinical studies need a permanently assigned statistician, not only during protocol design and during the final evaluation. Therefore, the statistician should be a member of the cooperative group performing the study and should follow the study throughout its course.

2. Medical Data Administrator

In Germany, since 1969 we are lucky to have a new profession, specially trained, with a three-year training program in medicine, mathematics and statistics, documentation, EDP, and organization. The Medical Data Administrator handles the following tasks in clinical studies ("his-or-her studies"): design, drawing, and distribution of the forms, randomization according to the stratified plan, checking and filing the records, reminding the units about overdue records, correcting data after clarifying questionable points with the clinical units, developing drug classifications, coding the forms, supervising the keypunching, loading the computer with the data, and all the computer work for the evaluation.

Both the statistician and his Medical Data Administrator must monitor a cooperative multicenter study at all times while the study is being conducted. These are some of the experiences of the Gnotobiotic Project Group.

4

Survival Studies Using a Computer-Based Hospital Registry of 29,000 Cancer Patients

M. K. Palmer

Christie Hospital and
Holt Radium Institute
Manchester
Great Britain

WHAT DO WE KNOW ABOUT the survival of patients with cancer? There are four main sources of information.

1. Mortality statistics
2. Regional cancer registries
3. Randomized clinical trials
4. Large cancer hospitals serving a region

Mortality statistics are of limited value in survival studies of cancer patients. Certified causes of death are often inaccurate, and, although population coverage is complete, the numbers of registrations of new cases to which they must be related are often incomplete. Moreover, mortality in one year is related to incidence in previous years, up to a decade or more.

So far as British Regional Cancer Registries are concerned, few record important prognostic information such as stage of disease, while the inclusion of registrations from non-specialist hospitals and family doctors increases the number of errors in important items such as site of disease and histological type. The extent of follow-up information collected also varies among registries.

Patients entered into clinical trials are always a select group, their work-up is usually much more detailed than would be the case otherwise, and their numbers are often small. Therefore their survival patterns are probably different from that of patients with the same type of disease in the general population.

Survival information from large, specialist centers, where the quality of data is often very good and the extent of follow-up virtually complete, has been relatively neglected.

In this chapter, I wish to describe the way in which data routinely recorded at the Christie Hospital and Holt Radium Institute in Manchester, England, can be used to produce survival curves of patients treated for cancer and to identify factors which influence survival.

The Christie Hospital provides a centralized radiotherapy service to a population of almost five million in the northwest part of England. About 6,000 new patients with cancer are registered annually; this is about 40% of all patients in the region, but for some cancer sites, such as the uterine cervix, larynx, pharynx, mouth, and testes, where the preference throughout the region is to treat with X-rays, the referral percentages are much greater: between 80 and 95%.

Information on the 29,000 patients registered between 1968 and 1973 is held on computer. The information for each patient consists of (1) identification data, that is, registration number, age, and sex; (2) the site of any previous malignancy; and (3) diagnostic information—this includes the site of the present malignancy, its stage, the sites of any metastases, histology reports, and the treatment given. Five-year follow-up information for patients treated in the years 1968–1971 has recently been added to the main data file; this information includes whether death was from a cause completely unrelated to the cancer for which treatment was initially given.

A lot of care is taken to maintain the accuracy of these records. The clerical staff reads through each patient's case notes very carefully, and these are returned to the doctor in charge if any information is missing or inconsistent. As a further check a computer program subjects each coded record to 56 detailed validations: rejected records are added to the main data file, but only after they have been corrected.

So, we now have available for survival studies a large volume of accurate data, routinely collected, on all patients referred to the hospital. In addition to this I would mention that there are many studies and clinical trials in which much more detailed information is recorded for smaller groups of patients with particular types of cancer, but it is the use of the routinely recorded data that I want to describe. This information is being used in two ways.

1. To monitor survival of cancer patients
2. To identify prognostic factors.

The intention is to produce regular reports showing the survival of patients categorized by site, histological type, stage, and treatment. Comparison of reports for different years will reveal whether changes in survival have occurred. The computer programs to produce these reports are nearing completion; the statistical problems of monitoring survival in this way have yet to be examined.

The identification of factors which influence survival is, of course, restricted to those items which have been routinely coded, but nevertheless worthwhile analyses can be carried out. An example, using data on 447 patients with cancer of the mouth who were treated at the Christie Hospital in the four years 1968–1971, will now be presented. These patients

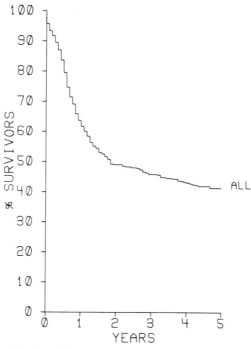

Fig. 1. Christie Hospital and Holt Radium Institute: Survival of 447 patients with mouth cancer, treated 1968–71

comprised some 85% of all patients with mouth cancer in the region, so I don't think the results can be too unrepresentative of survival of mouth cancer patients in general.

A decision-table processing language, FILETAB, was used to select these cases and list survival times and values of covariates. This was then the input to a survival analysis program. Figure 1 shows the survival of the entire group of patients.

A very useful facility we have is that, after carrying out the necessary calculations, the computer draws the axes, labels, and curves on an X–Y plotter. This can then be photographed directly by the Medical Illustration Department, who prepare the slides. In the process of calculating these curves, patients alive at the time that follow-up was coded were given censored survival times. Patients who had died of completely unrelated causes also were given censored times. Other patients, for whom the cause of death was or may have been mouth cancer, had exact survival times.

What factors may affect survival of patients with mouth cancer? Here, age groups <50 years, 50–59, 60–69, 70–79, and 80+ have been defined, and Figure 2 shows the survival in each group. Clearly the deterioration in survival with increasing age of the patient is very steep, and this trend is statistically highly significant.

Table I shows the number of patients, the number of deaths observed, and the total exposure to risk of death in each age group. The relative death rate in the eldest group is almost three times that in the youngest age group. (The relative death rate is the ratio O/E, and this will be 1 if survival in the subgroup is about average for the group as a whole.) And $p = 0.0001$ on a logrank test.

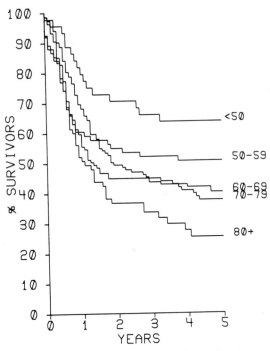

Fig. 2.   Christie Hospital and Holt Radium Institute: Survival of 447 patients with mouth cancer, treated 1968–71

Figure 3 shows that the stage of disease also has a very marked effect. These patients were staged according to the system in use at the Christie Hospital, which differs from the UICC 1974 stage-grouping recommendations, mainly between stages 3 and 4. The relative death rate is about four times greater in patients with stage 4 than stage 1 disease, and the trend is statistically highly significant, $p = 0.0006$. (see Table II).

On the other hand, it is seen in Figure 4 that there is no statistically significant difference

TABLE I[a]

Age	No. of patients	Deaths observed (O)	Exposure (E)	Relative death rate (O/E)
<50	44	20	35	0.58
50–59	74	37	46	0.81
60–69	134	81	83	0.98
70–79	120	75	65	1.15
80+	75	53	38	1.41

[a] Chi-square (trend) = 15.94, 1 df, $p = 0.0001$.

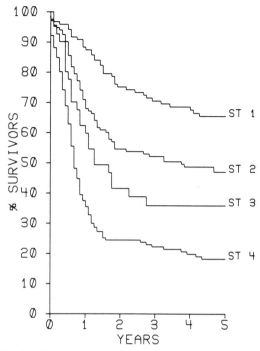

Fig. 3. Christie Hospital and Holt Radium Institute: Survival of 447 patients with mouth cancer, treated 1968–71

in survival between the sexes, and Table III shows that the relative death rates are 1.05 and 0.94, and $p = 0.40$.

Great care is taken in coding, as accurately as possible, the site of the cancer within the mouth. For large tumors this is the site of origin or main bulk of the tumor. Figure 5 shows survival according to site within the mouth. The sites are *cheek*, *gum* or *alveolus* (upper and lower combined), *floor*, *hard palate*, and *anterior two-thirds of the tongue*. The anatomical definition of *mouth* and the sites within the mouth conform to the UICC 1974

TABLE II[a]

Stage	No. of patients	Deaths observed (O)	Exposure (E)	Relative death rate (O/E)
1	122	45	113	0.40
2	132	71	104	0.68
3	41	26	27	0.96
4	151	124	72	1.71

[a] Chi-square (trend) = 11.69, 1 df, $p = 0.006$.

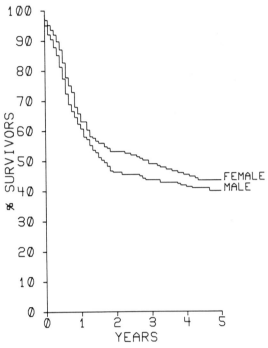

Fig. 4. Christie Hospital and Holt Radium Institute: Survival of 447 patients with mouth cancer, treated 1968–71

recommendations. Survival of patients with cancer of the tongue appears worse, but Table IV shows that the relative death rates vary only between 0.88 for cheek and 1.17 for tongue, and the difference in survival between the sites is not statistically significant. It was found however that patients with cancer arising in the anterior tongue tended to be slightly younger and to have somewhat less extensive disease than patients with cancer of other parts of the mouth, and patients with gum cancer tended to have more extensive disease. In order to examine the effect of the site of the disease on survival, independent of the concomitant effects of stage and age, 20 strata were defined by the combinations of 4 stages and 5 age groups. O and E values were calculated within each strata and summed over all strata to produce an adjusted table (see Table V) of relative death rates.

TABLE III

Sex	No. of patients	Deaths observed (O)	Exposure (E)	Relative death rate (O/E)
Males	262	157	150	1.05
Females	185	109	116	0.94

[a] Chi-square = 0.69, 1 df, p = 0.40.

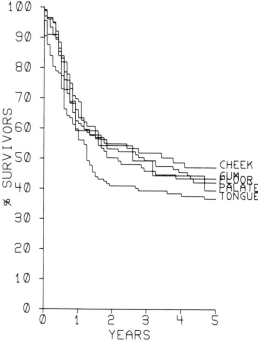

Fig. 5. Christie Hospital and Holt Radium Institute: Survival of 447 patients with mouth cancer, treated 1968–71

The order of sites from best to worst survival is very similar, but the difference is now statistically highly significant. The survival of patients with carcinoma of the tongue is seen to be relatively much worse, while that of patients with cancer of the gum improved slightly. So here we can say that the precise location of the tumor within the mouth is yet another prognostic factor, as well as the stage of disease and the age of the patient.

TABLE IV[a]

Site	No. of patients	Deaths observed (O)	Exposure (E)	Relative death rate (O/E)
Cheek	75	41	46	0.88
Gum	113	65	69	0.94
Floor	100	59	62	0.95
Palate	22	14	14	1.00
Tongue	137	87	74	1.17

[a] Chi-square = 3.26, 4 df, p = 0.52.

TABLE V[a,b]

Site	No. of patients	Deaths observed (O)	Adjusted exposure (E)	Adjusted R.D.R. (O/E)	Unadjusted R.D.R. (O/E)
Gum	113	65	87	0.75	0.94
Floor	100	58	67	0.87	0.95
Cheek	75	41	42	0.98	0.88
Palate	22	14	14	1.00	1.00
Tongue	137	87	55	1.57	1.17

[a] Chi-square = 30.30, 4 df, p = 0.0000.

Finally then, the existence of a large volume of accurate data on all patients registered at a large radiotherapy center provides us with the opportunity to calculate survival curves for any group of patients defined by site of disease, stage, age, sex, histological type, or treatment. This information can be used to monitor trends in survival over many years and complements the more detailed information that is recorded for patients in clinical trials and other studies. Also, the example I have demonstrated shows how these routinely collected data can be used to identify factors that influence prognosis of patients with cancer.

CHAPTER

5

Controlled Clinical Trials and the Importance of Medical Judgment

R. Burkhardt and G. Kienle

Gemeinnütziges Gemeinschaftskrankenhaus
Herdecke
West Germany

IN THE FEDERAL REPUBLIC OF GERMANY, a new drug law came into effect at the beginning of 1978. Now, as a result of long and difficult discussions, the law does not demand controlled clinical trials as qualification for the recognition and registration of drugs. In the official report of the Parliamentary Committee, which was responsible for the final version of the law, it was stated that a "decision-theory" approach would be adequate for the admission of drugs, and that such decisions might be based on more or less clear evidence for the efficacy of the respective drug. Moreover, the law provides for commissions to regulate the admission of drugs; these commissions are to include physicians, pharmacists, pharmacologists, and statisticians. All members of these commissions have to be experts in special pharmaceutical fields. In short, the legislators have made decisions concerning drug regulation a question of individual judgment, which need not be based on the results of controlled clinical trials.

To understand this development, it is necessary to make a clear distinction between theoretical ideas on the value of controlled experiments in the presence of random variations on the one hand, and the concrete environmental conditions in which clinical trials are carried out in practice on the other hand. From a theoretical point of view, controlled experiments based on random sampling are the most valuable tool we have to make inferences about parent populations. In practice, however, serious difficulties arise. They are partly of a methodological and partly of an ethical or legal nature.

As to the methodological difficulties, an excellent review is given in the book *Clinical Biostatistics* by Feinstein.[1] For instance, random sampling in fact almost never takes place in controlled clinical trials. The opposite is the case. Patients come to a particular clinic for specific reasons, and the further selection for a trial taking place is no random process. Therefore, all statistical tests based on random sampling (and this is the absolute majority of tests) are used in the absence of an essential prerequisite for their application. From the point of view of medical reality, we should refrain from drawing statistical inferences from "random" samples to parent populations and instead confine ourselves to statistical statements on the result of the trials, for instance by using permutation tests.

The list of such fundamental problems could easily be extended; the interested reader is referred to Feinstein.[1] In addition, there are many practical problems, which is why we have good and bad controlled clinical trials. Consequently, readers of publications about the results of controlled trials have to judge their value and estimate to what extent the results can be transferred to other patients. This estimation is clearly also a medical judgment. It is exactly for this reason that the German parliament introduced drug registration commissions to make decisions about the proposed admission of drugs on the basis of medical judgments about the real significance of the submitted investigations.

Let us now turn to ethical considerations. A lot of papers have been published on this subject. Sir Austin Bradford Hill[2] stated in 1963 that one has to face the reality that controlled randomized trials can only be performed with patients to whom the doctor believes the treatments being compared in the trial to be a matter of indifference. "By certain omissions from a trial we may limit the generality of the answer given by it, but on ethical grounds that must be accepted." [2] If two drugs seem to be very different at the beginning of a trial, it might be impossible to find patients for whom "treatment indifference" would exist, and therefore the trial cannot be carried out. In 1976 Byar et al.[3] discussed the situation where patients have already entered the study: "Whenever a physician thinks that the interests of his patient are at stake, he must be free to treat the patient as he sees fit. . . . Even though allowing patients to be withdrawn from the study may greatly complicate the analysis of the data, it is an absolutely essential requirement for an ethically conducted trial."

Consequently, in numerous cases doctors thought it impossible to perform controlled trials, in many other cases patients were withdrawn, or, in extreme cases, trials were completely stopped—all this on the basis of medical judgment.

In Germany, this problem is now being reconsidered from the point of view of criminal law. This development was started by a book by Professor Fincke,[4] who investigated the legal implications of controlled clinical trials. He is Professor of Criminal Law at the University of Bielefeld. In his book Professor Fincke discusses a hypothetical case. He assumes that a new drug against cancer has been developed which in uncontrolled treatment appeared to be highly effective. Then a controlled multicenter trial is performed with a standard treatment serving as control. Each group consists of 1,000 patients. In the group treated with the new drug, 500 patients died within a certain period, and in the control group there are 700 deaths within this period. The difference is statistically significant.

Fincke comes to the conclusion that the doctors who participated in the trial and who shared the opinion that the new drug seemed to be highly effective were guilty of deliberate homicide. This legal conclusion can clearly be seen as arising from the ethical considerations mentioned by Hill.[2] But Fincke extends his result to situations where at the beginning of the trial the doctors judge the drugs being compared to be equivalent. After studying several publications on controlled clinical trials where mortality served as a measure for efficacy and where the differences between the mortality rates were statistically significant, he found his conclusion to be valid for these situations also. So the statistician must ask himself if there are plausible reasons for this extension.

To answer this question it is useful to differentiate between ethics of individual benefit and ethics of group benefit. Lellouch and Schwartz,[5] in a study published in 1971, reported on the results of some computer simulations to compare the effectiveness of therapeutic trials based on ethics of group benefit with trials based on ethics of individual benefit (using a Bayesian approach). They stated that Neyman-Pearson statistics include ethics of group benefit when applied to medicine. Statistically significant differences in mortality as a basis for the decision concerning which drug to apply for the benefit of future patients can only be obtained from sufficiently different rates of mortality in the groups to be compared in the trial. Some patients in the trial must be given (more or less consciously) the less effective treatment, and must therefore die, in order to find out how to treat future patients with maximum benefit.

The limitations that Hill and Byar consider necessary result from ethics of individual benefit. Thereby they implicitly admit the existence of a tendency against individual benefit or, positively, a tendency towards group benefit in controlled clinical trials. But it is difficult to understand how to get valid results if the point of view of individual benefit is taken seriously. For instance, towards the end of sequential medical trials there may arise the following situation, described by Lellouch and Schwartz:[5] "Towards the end of the trial, the path runs very near the borderline, which means that one of the two patients of each of the last pairs necessary to conclude the trial will receive a treatment which at that moment appears to be less effective than the other."

In principle, the same is true—though less apparent—for fixed-sample-size trials. It is common practice to do interim analyses (in Dr. Hill's paper this is again confirmed), even at the cost of obscuring the significance levels. According to Chalmers et al.[6] "the only known way to avoid the ethical . . . problem is to design studies so that the results are . . . closely monitored by peers who can advise the investigators when to stop the study . . . The mechanism adopted by the investigator . . . should be explained to the patient as part of the informed-consent procedure." Here the supervision of the data is recommended for ethical reasons, against the principles of statistical inference in fixed-sample-size trials.

When applying individual ethics, it might be impossible to finish studies that would show the superiority of a particular treatment. It might only be possible to conduct and finish studies that show as a result no difference between the treatments compared. Fortunately, in an unpublished paper Professor Fincke provides a legal solution for this problem; he differentiates between a contract for treatment and a contract for experimentation. Controlled clinical trials intended to show the superiority of a certain drug are prohibited by criminal law only in the first case, if there is a contract for treatment. In the second case, the patient is aware that he is to participate in a study in which he might receive a treatment which the doctor judges to be inferior to another treatment, and that he might die for this reason. If in spite of this he is willing to undergo this risk (possibly for a certain remuneration or, if he is an idealist, for the sake of future patients), the doctor is not obliged to use the therapy he considers to be best for this patient, but he can use the therapy that results from the randomization scheme.

The situation can be summarized as follows: In controlled clinical trials, conflicts may arise between individual and collective ethics. It is well known that the Declaration of Helsinki, as revised in Tokyo, supports the aspect of individual benefit. If Fincke is right, the same is true for German criminal law, if applied to clinical trials as they are usually conducted. Whether a trial can be conducted in the usual way, or whether it cannot be conducted at all, or only on the basis of a contract for experimentation, depends on the judgment of the doctors who are to participate in the trial. According to Fincke, the doctors are not allowed to retreat behind a pose of scientific ignorance. What counts in the legal sense is their personal estimation of the value of the drugs. It must be recognized that a doctor's indifference with regard to two particular drugs implies a personal estimation or, in other words, a medical judgment.

It is quite clear that medical ethics, that is to say individual ethics, and especially criminal law are of greater importance than scientific demands. So if conflicts arise (on the basis of medical judgment) they must clearly be decided in favor of medical ethics and law. This seems to be self-evident, but according to Fincke it is frequently violated in practice.

Now some comments on the papers presented by Dr. Byar and Dr. Zelen. Dr. Byar gave a list of the principal advantages of randomized trials. One point in his list is that the results of randomized trials are more likely to be convincing than comparisons with historical controls.

Other people are more likely to be convinced if there is sufficient evidence for efficacy or superiority of a given drug. The more evidence, the more convincing are the results. Applied to mortality rates that means the higher the difference in the mortality rates, the higher the evidence and the greater likelihood of convincing other persons. In short, convincing others will depend on more or less significant differences of death rates in the trials. Moreover, the concept of convincing other persons implies that the investigator who undertakes the trial may be convinced earlier than other people, and that in order to convince others, he must continue the randomized trial beyond his personal convinction. Convincing others is especially important when the other persons belong to drug administrations. Drug administrations clearly represent the point of view of collective ethics. So we see the conflict here again.

The second interesting point in Dr. Byar's list is that randomized trials may be more ethical than the use of historical controls, since fewer patients need be treated to get a convincing answer. The motivation can be acknowledged, but overlooked is the fact that patients may be treated against the personal conviction of the doctor—that means against individual ethics and, if Fincke is right, against the law. If the ethical responsibility is transferred to ethical committees or advisory boards, the conflict will arise there.

An important point is the informed consent. In Fincke's terms the question is whether an informed consent means that a contract for experimentation has been settled. Fincke disagrees and says that such a contract has to be settled explicitly.

In his paper, Dr. Zelen proposed randomization of the consent. This does not change the situation, for patients in group G1 ("do not seek consent") automatically will receive treatment A without regard to the personal judgment of the doctors. The problem is to find a randomization scheme that is in accordance with ethics of individual benefit, but this is surely impossible.

REFERENCES

1. Feinstein, Alvan R. (1977). *Clinical Biostatistics*, The C. V. Mosby Company, Saint Louis.

2. Hill, Austin Bradford (1963). Medical ethics and controlled trials. *Br Med* 1043–49.

3. Byar, David P., et al. (1976). Randomized clinical trials. *New England J Med*, 74–80.

4. Fincke, Martin (1977). *Arzneimittelprüfung—Strafbare Versuchsmethoden*, C. F. Müller Juristischer Verlag, Heidelberg, Karlsruhe.

5. Lellouch, J. and Schwartz, D. (1971). L'essai thérapeutique: éthique individuelle ou éthique collective? *Rev Inst Int Stat*, **39**: 127–36.

6. Chalmers, Thomas C. et al. (1972). Controlled studies in clinical cancer research. *N Engl J Med*, **287**: 75–78.

6

Heterogeneity and Standardization in Clinical Trials

Richard Simon

Division of Cancer Treatment
National Cancer Institute
Bethesda, Maryland 20014

1. INTRODUCTION

CLINICAL TRIALS ARE characterized by heterogeneity in the patients treated and variability in the responses obtained. It is because of such heterogeneity that statistics assumes an important role in the conduct of these studies. In fields where response is completely predictable without variability, there is little need for statistical design or analysis. In this chapter I will try to review some methods for dealing with patient heterogeneity.

2. COMPARABILITY AND RANDOMIZATION

One basic approach consists of restricting the study to patients within major disease categories, e.g., defined by site, stage or histology, and trying to achieve comparability among the treatment groups with regard to other factors thought to affect response. Comparability denotes equal heterogeneity, and complete comparability with regard to all factors is conceptually unachievable. There are often many such factors, and important ones are generally either unknown or unmeasurable. Though a reasonably good degree of comparability with regard to major known prognostic factors is important, extreme efforts to achieve comparability with regard to all variables suspected of influencing response can interfere with the successful application of other methods for dealing with heterogeneity. I will say more about this later.

While we are on this topic, however, the relationship between comparability and randomization should be mentioned. Basic objectives of statistical design and analysis in comparative studies include obtaining an unbiased estimate of the difference in efficacy of the treatments and determination of the precision of this estimate. Randomization does not ensure comparability of treatment groups with regard to prognostic factors that are known and measured any better than does matching, using historical controls; in fact, it may do worse. This fact is sometimes used spuriously as an argument against randomization. Randomization also does not ensure that the treatment groups will be comparable with regard to unknown prognostic factors. There is no way of ensuring this other than to perform studies that increase our knowledge of such factors. Randomization does, however, ensure that the totality of uncontrollable sources of variability and noncomparability will have a symmetric and known distribution among the treatment groups. Practically, this means that there is no systematic bias resulting from such things as subjectivity in the assignment of treatments or from unknown time trends or changes in referral patterns. It also means that if the number of patients treated is sufficiently large, the estimator of treatment difference will be an accurate reflection of the true relative benefit of one treatment compared to the other. The second important consequence of randomization is that the precision of the estimator of treatment difference is known; thus confidence limits and significance levels can be calculated. Without randomization, one must assume, and hope, that the groups being compared can be treated as if they have identically distributed realizations of unknown prognostic factors. Such an assumption is implicit in the use of regression models to evaluate a current treatment with historical controls. In such studies, where there is noncomparability of known prognostic factors that must be adjusted for, the assumption that the unknown prognostic factors are identically distributed among the treatment groups seems quite questionable.

3. STRATIFICATION

I shall now turn to the topic of stratification in randomized clinical trials. Stratification usually denotes partitioning the patients into mutually exclusive subsets based upon pretreatment characteristics thought to affect prognosis. For example, as shown in Figure 1, in a comparison of treatments for testicular cancer, the factors may be histology and stage.

| | Stage | |
	II	III
Teratocarcinoma with or without seminoma		
Embryonal carcinoma with or without seminoma		
Either of above with elements of choriocarcinoma		

Fig. 1   Design for stratified randomization in testicular cancer.

AAABBB	BBBAAA
AABABB	BBABAA
AABBAB	BBAABA
AABBBA	BBAAAB
ABAABB	BABBAA
ABABAB	BABABA
ABABBA	BABAAB
ABAAAB	BAABBA
ABBABA	BAABAB
ABBBAA	BAAABB

Fig. 2   Permuted blocks of length 6 for two treatments.

These two stratification factors here define six subsets. Within each subset, or stratum, a pseudorandomization is performed. One kind of pseudorandomization is the permuted block design shown in Figure 2. A permuted block of length 6 for two treatments, A and B, is a sequence of three As and three Bs. In general for two treatments, a permuted block of length $2k$ is a sequence of As and Bs containing exactly kAs and kBs. The 20 possible permuted blocks of length 6 are shown in Figure 2. The treatment assignment is determined by a succession of randomly selected permuted blocks within each stratum. If there are three treatments, permuted blocks of k instances of each of three letters are used. Generally, the permuted blocks of distinct strata are prepared independently of each other. If stratification is to be employed, a pseudorandom mechanism such as permuted blocks is necessary, because pure randomization within each stratum is equivalent to no stratification at all.

Stratification is generally used to ensure a greater degree of comparability of the treatment groups with regard to known prognostic factors than can be obtained by pure randomization. When feasible, it is often desirable to incorporate the stratification factors into the analysis, in order to increase the sensitivity of the trial. It is general practice to stratify and then ignore the stratification factors in the analysis. This results in a more precise estimator of treatment differences than if stratification were not employed, because the estimator is not subject to the fluctuations caused by variable degrees of imbalance with regard to known factors. A defect of ignoring stratification factors in the analysis, however, is that the precision of the estimator of treatment difference will be better than that calculated from the data. Treating the known sources of variability embodied in the stratification factors as unknown sources of noise is to be avoided when possible. To help clarify this point, consider the illustration in Figure 3. It is assumed that there are two strata and two treatments. The upper graph depicts the frequency function, or histogram, of survival for each of the two treatment groups within each of the two stratum. For purposes of illustration, the concept of censored survivals is ignored. It is clear that stratum II patients have a better prognosis than stratum I patients, because their frequency functions are displaced to the right. Also, within each stratum treatment B seems more effective than treatment A. The desirable analysis consists of calculating an estimate Δ_I of the treatment difference within stratum I and an estimate Δ_{II} of the treatment difference within stratum II. A weighted average of Δ_I and Δ_{II} is used as the overall test statistic for evaluating the statistical significance of the treatment dif-

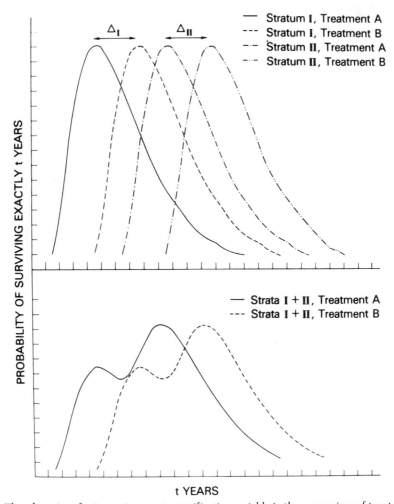

Fig. 3   The advantage of using an important stratification variable in the comparison of two treatments.

ference. Of course significance tests could be performed within each stratum, but the limited number of patients usually makes this undesirable because the power of the test will be small. The variability associated with the weighted average of Δ_I and Δ_{II} is estimated based upon the variability for each of four curves at the top of Figure 3. The treatment differences in the case shown are reasonably large relative to the variability of the individual curves, so if the number of patients is not too small, a statistically significant result will be declared.

The bottom illustration is intended to represent a redrawing of the top illustration, except that the stratum distinctions are ignored. Each of the two curves represents a frequency function of survival for a pooled treatment group consisting of patients from both strata. Though the two treatment groups may be perfectly "comparable" with regard to the stratification variable, if the pooled groups are compared directly a very weak significance test will result. Thus, when important stratification variables can be incoporated into the

Histology

	Stage II		Stage III	
	Age<15	Age≥15	Age<15	Age≥15
Teratocarcinoma	A✓	A✓	A✓	B✓
	A✓	A✓	A✓	A✓
	B	A✓	A✓	A✓
	A	B	B	B
	B	B	B	B
	B	B	B	A
Embryonal Carcinoma	A✓	B	B✓	A✓
	A✓	B	B✓	B✓
	B	A	A	B✓
	B	A	A	B✓
	B	A	B	A
	A	B	A	A
Terato or Embryonal Carcinoma with Elements or Choriocarcinoma	B✓	B	A✓	B✓
	B	A	B✓	B✓
	A	A	B✓	A
	A	B	B✓	A
	B	B	A	A
	A	A	A	B

		A	B
Histology:	Teratocarcinoma	10	1
	Embryonal Carcinoma	3	5
	Elements of Choriocarcinoma	1	6
Stage:	II	7	1
	III	7	11
Age:	<15	8	6
	≥15	6	6
		14	12

Fig. 4   Imbalances in an overstratified design.

analysis, we are in a sense eliminating the random fluctuations caused by such variables in our comparison of treatments.

Though limited stratification is desirable, overstratification can be detrimental to a trial. With numerous strata, many of them may contain only a single patient at the conclusion of the trial and many strata will not contain enough patients to complete the first permuted block. Consequently, balance with regard to the most important factors may be impaired by the inclusion of secondary factors into the design. Even the total number of patients assigned to each treatment may be unbalanced. Overstratification in the extreme becomes equivalent to no stratification.[1] To illustrate this point consider Figure 4. The sequence of treatment assignments is generated for the stratification design shown previously, with age as an additional factor. The sequence of treatments results from independently and randomly selecting permuted blocks of length 6 for two treatments, A and B. The check marks indicate the treatment assignments and distribution of stratification factors for the first 26 patients. Although the sizes of the treatment groups are well balanced in this case, 14 As to 12 Bs, the distributions of histology and stage are quite unbalanced, as shown at the bottom of the figure. This results from having too few patients for the number of strata and block length used. In this particular case, the problem could perhaps be solved by using shorter blocks, blocks of 2 or 4. In general, however, even if blocks of length 2 are used, if the degree of stratification is too great, the same problem will result.

From a more statistical point of view, the problem of overstratification is not just one of comparability with regard to the marginal distributions of the stratification variables. As mentioned, it is desirable to utilize stratification factors in the analysis in order to determine correctly the precision of the estimator of treatment difference. The most desirable method of performing an overall significance test is to determine an estimate of treatment difference within each stratum and to use as the test statistic a weighted average of these within-stratum estimates. Overstratification causes two problems in this analysis. First, strata which only contain patients assigned to one of the treatments contribute nothing to the analysis, because no within-stratum estimate of treatment difference can be determined. Second, even though a stratum may contain patients of both treatment groups, if the within-stratum sample sizes are too greatly reduced by the inclusion of variables of secondary importance, the statistical power of the stratified analysis decreases. Because of this, one is forced either to ignore stratification factors in the analysis or to pool strata. Even with simple pooling of strata, the estimator of the variance of treatment difference may be inflated by the attempt to balance the treatment groups by factors not included in the analysis. Often, the ignored stratification factors are of little importance anyway, and the inflation of the variance will be minimal. Luck may fail, however, and the pooling of strata may not result in superstrata that are well balanced among the treatments for purposes of analysis.

Several individuals—Harville,[2] Taves,[3] and Pocock and Simon[1]—have studied adaptive stratification designs. With these methods, the treatment assigned to a patient depends upon the levels of the stratification factors for patients who have previously entered the trial. By using this information, it is possible to effectively ensure that the treatment groups are well balanced with regard to the marginal distribution of many stratification variables. For small studies of diseases, in which many factors are thought to influence prognosis, these methods are of value. The methods, or simplified versions of them, are also of value for incorporating *institution* as a stratification variable in studies with many institutions and other stratification variables. Generally, where such procedures are used there are too many stratification variables, or a variable such as *institution* has too many levels, to be incorporated in the analysis. The method is used to ensure marginal comparability of the treatment groups at the price of potentially reduced statistical power. In many situations, the stratification variables are not really as important as they are thought to be. Hence, obtaining marginal comparability gives confidence in the result, while ignoring the variables in the analysis produces no serious loss in statistical power. A limitation of adaptive stratification methods, however, is their logistical complexity. Since the treatment assignment for a patient depends upon the levels of the stratification factors for previously entered patients, the sequence of treatment assignments cannot be prespecified at the start of the trial. Zelen[4] has developed a method of this type for dealing fairly simply with *institution* as a stratification variable. In general, however, it is necessary to use a computer or programmable calculator for each patient being randomized. A computer printout of the next treatment assignment may be maintained for the next patient in each possible stratum. When a request for a treatment assignment occurs, it is immediately satisfied. Then the file is updated and the computer printout for all possible "next patients" is obtained. Friedman and White[5] have shown that the method of Pocock and Simon can be employed in a workable, though deterministic, manner without the use of a computer.

4. ADJUSTMENT PROCEDURES

In an extensive paper on clinical trials, Peto et al.[6] dismiss stratification for all but small studies. They view it as a complication rendered unnecessary by the development of methods of analysis that adjust for prognostic factors. This theme was repeated in an editorial in the *British Medical Journal*: "Nowadays it is generally unnecessary to randomize patients within separate groups according to prognostic factors, since these are better allowed for retrospectively in the analysis."[7]

I have already described in general terms a class of adjustment procedures to be used in conjunction with stratification. These procedures consist of determining an estimator of within-stratum treatment difference and using a weighted average of these estimators as the test statistic. Pairing of observations is the simplest example of such a procedure. The commonly used Mantel-Haenszel test[8] can also be employed in this manner for comparing response rates, survival curves, or remission-duration curves. Such procedures are specific instances of a broader class of regression models. The usual linear regression model with normally distributed errors finds limited applications for therapeutic clinical trials in oncology. One regression method that is widely used for analysis of survival or remission duration data will be described in order to give a feel for such procedures.

The proportional hazards model for analyzing survival or remission duration curves can be defined as follows[9]:

$$\lambda(t\,|\,\mathbf{x}) = f(t)\exp(\beta_1 x_1 + \beta_2 x_2 + \ldots + \beta_n x_n)$$

The notation $\mathbf{x}$ denotes a vector of prognostic variables having components $x_1, x_2, \ldots x_n$. The function $\lambda(t\,|\,\mathbf{x})$ represents the force of mortality for a patient having characteristics described by the vector $\mathbf{x}$. It can be thought of as the probability of death at time t for such a patient alive just before t. This function $\lambda(t\,|\,\mathbf{x})$ is called the hazard function of a survival distribution. In the above model, the hazard function for a patient equals some unknown function of time, $f(t)$, times an exponential function that depends upon the patient characteristics $x_1, x_2, \ldots, x_n$ and upon unknown regression coefficients $\beta_1, \beta_2, \ldots, \beta_n$, but not upon t. This model is called the proportional hazards model, because the unknown function of time is the same for each patient; that is, the ratio of hazards for two different patients

$$\frac{\lambda(t\,|\,\mathbf{x}^1)}{\lambda(t\,|\,\mathbf{x}^2)} = \frac{\exp(\beta_1 x_1{}^1 + \beta_2 x_2{}^1 + \ldots + \beta_n x_n{}^1)}{\exp(\beta_1 x_1{}^2 + \beta_2 x_2{}^2 + \ldots + \beta_n x_n{}^2)}$$

$$X_1 = \begin{cases} 1 & \text{if patient receives treatment A} \\ 0 & \text{if patient receives treatment B} \end{cases}$$

$$X_2 = \text{Age in years}$$

$$X_3 = \text{Karnofsky performance score}$$

$$X_4 = \begin{cases} 1 & \text{if patient has visceral dominant disease} \\ 0 & \text{otherwise} \end{cases}$$

$$X_5 = \begin{cases} 1 & \text{if patient has osseous dominant disease} \\ 0 & \text{otherwise} \end{cases}$$

Fig. 5 One method of defining variables for use with an adjustment procedure.

is independent of time. This result is of great statistical importance, because it implies that the regression coefficients can be estimated and their significance tested without knowledge of or assumptions about the function $f(t)$. For example, one need not assume that the underlying distribution is exponential.

To use this model in analysis, it must be decided what variables to include. One example of the use of this model is shown in Figure 5. In the context of therapeutic studies, such methods are called adjustment procedures, because the treatment effect β_1 is estimated and its significance tested after adjustment for the effects of the patient characteristics. There are difficulties, however, associated with defining variables as in Figure 5. First, it is assumed that if age has an effect ($\beta_2 \neq 0$), then the logarithm of the hazard function for a 50-year-old patient is twice that of a similar 25-year-old. A similar assumption is made by the manner in which Karnofsky performance status is included. The second difficulty in defining variables as in Figure 5 is that the effect of the variables is assumed to be linearly additive on the logarithm of the hazard function. These are all assumptions that should be avoided without a test of their validity. These assumptions can be avoided by defining the variables, as in Figure 6. The evaluation of treatment effect based on defining variables in this way is performed by estimating β_{13} and testing whether it is significantly different from zero.

Peto et al.[6] point out that adjustment methods can be used regardless of whether or not stratification was performed in treatment assignment. They grant that stratification does help ensure that the stratification factors will be well distributed among the treatment groups so that a powerful statistical test will result, but they argue that for large clinical trials the expected power, even without stratification, will be nearly as good. Mantel has emphasized that the use of stratification in treatment assignment interferes with the flexible use of such adjustment procedures in the analysis, because, strictly speaking, all stratification factors must be included in the model.

Though these points are well taken, they are not entirely convincing with regard to small or moderate size clinical trials. For such studies some degree of stratification by important

1. Stratify the patients into 12 strata based on the characteristics:

$$Age \quad \leq 50 \quad versus \quad > 50$$

$$Performance\ Status \quad \leq 75 \quad versus \quad > 75$$

$$Dominant\ Site \quad visceral\ versus\ osseous\ versus\ soft\ tissue$$

2. Arbitrarily number the strata 1, 2,..., 12

3. Define

$$X_1 = \begin{cases} 1 & \text{if the patient is in stratum 1} \\ 0 & \text{otherwise} \end{cases}$$

$$X_2 = \begin{cases} 1 & \text{if the patient is in stratum 2} \\ 0 & \text{otherwise} \end{cases}$$

.
.
.

$$X_{12} = \begin{cases} 1 & \text{if the patient is in stratum 12} \\ 0 & \text{otherwise} \end{cases}$$

$$X_{13} = \begin{cases} 1 & \text{if the patient receives treatment A} \\ 0 & \text{if the patient receives treatment B} \end{cases}$$

Fig. 6   Use of indicator variables to define strata for an adjustment procedure.

variables does seem desirable. Also, the expected power of significance tests is not the only notion of power to be considered. Viewed in one way, stratification is an insurance policy against low probability imbalances that can ruin or severely decrease the sensitivity of a trial. Any particular trial will be performed only once, and if the treatment effect is nearly confounded with the effect of a prognostic factor, it will be little consolation to know that the expected power was adequate.[10] If the degree of stratification employed to obtain this insurance is too great to incorporate into the analysis, however, one must accept the price of potentially decreased statistical power. Though such insurance may seem unnecessary for the final analysis of large clinical trials, Zelen has pointed out that all large studies are of small or moderate size at some interim analyses.

The use of prospective stratification tends to avoid situations in which conclusions of a study are not convincing to the medical community because of suspicion and lack of understanding of an analysis used to adjust for a lack of comparability. Using stratification, the method of analysis may be the same and still not be widely understood, but it is less likely that a troublesome lack of comparability will exist to arouse suspicion.

Though I have spoken favorably of adjustment methods for the analysis of both stratified and unstratified studies, the validity of such techniques depends upon the adequacy of the assumed statistical model and upon large-sample approximations. For example, the proportional hazard model described makes the assumption that if the five-year survival rate for one group is zero than it is similarly zero for all other groups. This results because one distribution function is a power of the other. There may be ambiguity concerning which variables to adjust for and how they should be represented in the model. Adjustment for all variables may entail considerable loss of power, and selection of adjusting variables by stepwise procedures or informal methods results in an arbitrary conditional significance level. Too much flexibility in the selection of adjusting variables after the fact may result in the elimination of a real treatment difference or a critical dependence of the interpretation upon the selection of adjusting variables. Using pretreatment stratification, the adjusting variables and their discrete representations can be viewed as being uniquely determined by the design. Limited pretreatment stratification also ensures that interim analyses will be meaningful even though the sample sizes at that point may not be adequate for testing the adequacy of or utilizing an adjustment procedure.

It is true that some investigators give undue and detrimental emphasis to extensive stratification. Large definitive studies identifying which variables make important independent contributions to prognosis are very valuable. Such studies often demonstrate that potential stratification variables are so related that only a few should be included for design and analysis purposes, and that these few can play an important role in increasing the sensitivity of clinical trials.

5. GENERALIZATION OF CONCLUSIONS

If the conclusions of a clinical trial were not generalizable to patients other than those actually entered in the study, clinical research would be futile. The only statistical bias for generalization, however, is the assumption that the studied patients constitute a random sample from a larger population. Such random selection of patients is rarely if ever practiced, but in certain circumstances it is reasonable to generalize our conclusions as if our patients were so selected. For several aspects of study design now to be described, it is important to bear in mind the issue of generalization of conclusions.

The first such issue is the determination of patient eligibility requirements. Such requirements are generally based upon the expected ability of the patient to tolerate any of the treatments and that the potential benefits outweigh potential risks. Often such considerations do not uniquely define specific eligibility requirements, and there is discussion concerning whether various small, distinguishable subsets of patients should be included. One example of this occurs in chemotherapy studies that include subsets of more debilitated patients for whom it is planned beforehand to administer reduced doses. One must bear in mind that it will rarely be possible to compare treatment efficacy for such subgroups separately, because of limited sample sizes. The basic conclusion of the study will result from the overall comparison. Though the overall comparison may be balanced or adjusted for stratification factors, the conclusion based upon this comparison is generalizable only to a mixture of the same kinds of patients studied in the trial. The assumption that relative treatment efficacy is the same for all subgroups is rarely tenable. Consequently, it is important that the eligibility requirements define a medically meaningful set of patients, so that in reporting the results of the study a coherent statement can be made as to whom the conclusions apply. This point was emphasized by Sir A. B. Hill[11] in his description of a Medical Research Council trial of streptomycin: "In short, the questions asked of the trial were deliberately limited and these 'closely defined features were considered indispensable, for it was realized that no two patients have an identical form of the disease and it was desired to eliminate as many of the obvious variations as possible.' This planning . . . is a fundamental feature of the successful trial. To start out upon a trial with all and sundry included, and with the hope that the results can be sorted out statistically in the end is to court disaster."

Some statisticians today do not agree with this viewpoint, so strongly stated by Hill. They say, essentially, do not waste time arguing about whether subsets of patients should or should not be included in the trial; if it is reasonable to include them, then do so. One can evaluate at the conclusion of the trial whether the relative treatment efficacy differed among such subsets. For *very* large clinical trials, I believe that this viewpoint is reasonable. For intermediate size or small clinical trials, I believe that it provides fuel for erroneous conclusions based upon inadequate numbers, and adds considerable subjectivity to the analysis.

Similar considerations apply to two other important issues of study design. The first is standardization of surgery and radiotherapy in chemotherapy adjuvant studies. It is generally agreed that if we are studying the efficacy of chemotherapy, then administration of chemotherapy should be standardized. The question of standardization of the surgery or radiotherapy to which the chemotherapy is an adjuvant is somewhat more elusive. As just mentioned, if the local therapies are not standardized, then the conclusions apply, if at all, only to a mixture of patients receiving the same types of local therapy as those studied. This conclusion for mixed populations may in fact be valid for no specific patient. For example, chemotherapy may be beneficial to patients receiving extensive surgery with limited radiotherapy, but detrimental to patients receiving limited surgery with extensive radiotherapy. Because limited numbers of patients do not permit reliable evaluation of subsets, the variability introduced by nonstandardization makes the conclusion of no overall significant positive or negative effect of chemotherapy erroneous for all patients.

An additional issue of study design in which the above considerations apply is that of "collapsing the arms of a protocol." Consider for example the study schematic given in Figure 7. Patients are initially randomized to one of two possible induction treatments, *A* or *B*. Patients not achieving a complete remission go off study. Those who do achieve a complete remission are randomized to one of two possible maintenance treatments, *C* or *D*. If the efficacy of the induction agents is based only upon the proportion of complete remissions induced and upon toxicity during the induction phase, then the comparison of *A* and *B* is unaffected by the maintenance randomization. It is sometimes argued however that evaluation of the relative effects of *C* and *D* for maintaining remissions is unaffected by the induction randomization. That is, it is suggested that one can "collapse" the four

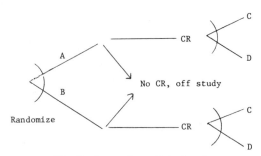

Fig. 7 A two-phase clinical trial.

arms of the protocol into two for comparing C and D, or that the induction treatment can be used as an adjusting variable in comparing the maintenance regimens. As previously described, this approach entails either (1) making the questionable assumption that the relative advantage or disadvantage of C versus D as a maintenance therapy does not depend upon which therapy is used for induction, (2) determining the sample size to be large enough to test this questionable assumption, or (3) having the conclusions apply "on the average." In this example, it is possible that maintenance C is cross-resistant with induction A but not B; whereas maintenance D is cross-resistant with induction B but not A. Unless the sample size is large enough to detect this reliably, the conclusion resulting from the comparison of C to D, for the mixture of patients receiving A and B, will be erroneous for all such individual patients.

The final issue to be mentioned in the context of generalizability of conclusions is that of patient disqualifications. Because we wish to evaluate treatment efficacy, we are tempted to disqualify patients who are not adequately treated for one reason or another. This is a very dangerous practice because of the potential bias it permits. In most situations, it is very unlikely that the patients who do not complete treatment can be realistically viewed as a random selection of all patients assigned that treatment. Generally, their prognoses are poor. Since the treatments being compared may differ in the kinds and quantities of potential disqualifications they produce, disqualifications based upon anything but eligibility criteria are very likely to introduce bias into the evaluation. The only fully reliable approach is to include in the analysis all eligible patients entered in the study. One is then evaluating the therapeutic *strategy* of attempting to administer treatment A versus the strategy of attempting to administer treatment B. The resulting conclusions may actually be more clinically relevant with regard to generalizations to broader patient populations.

REFERENCES

1. Pocock, S.J., and Simon, R. (1975). Sequential treatment assignment with balancing for prognostic factors in the controlled clinical trial. *Biometrics*, 31:103–15.

2. Harville, D.A. (1974). Nearly optimal allocation of experimental units using observed covariate values. *Technometric*, 16:589–99.

3. Taves, D.R. (1974). Minimization: A new method of assigning patients to treatment and control groups. *Clin Pharmacol Ther*, **15**:443–53.

4. Zelen, M. (1974). Randomization and stratification of patients to clinical trials. *J Chronic Dis*, **27**:365–75.

5. Freedman, L.S., and White, S.J. (1976). On the use of Pocock and Simon's method for balancing treatment numbers over prognostic factors in the controlled clinical trial. *Biometrics*, **32**:691–94.

6. Peto, R.; Pike, M.C.; Armitage, P.; et al. (1976). Design and analysis of randomized clinical trials requiring prolonged observation of each patient. I. Introduction and design. *Br J Cancer*, **34**:585–612.

7. Editorial (1977). Randomized clinical trials. *Br Med J*, **6071**:1238–39.

8. Mantel, M., and Haenszel, W. (1959). Statistical aspects of the analysis of data from retrospective studies of disease. *J Natl Cancer Inst*, **22**:719–48.

9. Cox, D.R. (1972). Regression models and life tables. *J Royal Statist Soc B*, **34**:187, 220.

10. Lasagna, L. (1955). Randomized clinical trials. *N Engl J Med*, **295**:1086–87.

11. Hill, A.B. (1951). The clinical trial. *Br Med Bull*, **7**:278–82.

7

Interim Analysis and Early Results in Clinical Trials

C. Hill and H. Sancho-Garnier

Institut Gustave Roussy
Villejuif, France

THE PROBLEM OF DOING interim analysis and giving publicity to early results of a trial through discussions and/or publications is a critical one in the conduct of a clinical trial. In a recent survey based on 50 randomly selected trials registered at the UICC information office, Stuart Pocock[5] found that 33 out of 40 answered "yes" to the question: "Was an interim analysis performed?" This confirms our experience that interim analysis is a very common practice.

We shall call *analysis* the study of any information about the trial, because the borderline between what is relevant to the comparison of the treatments and what is not is never clearly defined and indeed cannot be defined unequivocally. *Interim analysis* is an analysis performed before all the information that has been deemed necessary to ensure a certain power to the comparison has been assembled.

A general description of the state of the trial is the first step of any analysis. It enables one to:

1. watch the accrual rate center by center
2. check on the filling up of the forms
3. have regular descriptions of which patients are considered eligible or ineligible
4. check on the randomization process. Clinical trials conducted by clinicians still unfamiliar with the procedures involved show a tendency to drifting in the randomization process. By *drifting* we mean, for example, a situation where a patient is excluded after randomization, because the clinicians have decided *a posteriori* that the treatment randomly allocated to the patient is unsuitable.
5. study the reasons for postrandomization withdrawals
6. compare the actual treatments given to those decided upon in the protocol
7. help in following up the patients.

Sometimes a comparison between treatment groups is made of the distribution of characteristics of the patients involved. There are likely to be some differences, especially if many characteristics are tested. Such a comparison may detect drifting in the randomization process; this is the major reason for doing an analysis of randomly distributed patient characteristics.

The second step of the analysis consists of studying the results of the treatments as applied to the criteria defined in the protocol, such as: rate of early complication and side effects of treatment; tumor regression; recurrence or death rates; or any other measure.

The management of the trial should not be subject to discussion. It is a necessity and has not been given as much attention as it should have, perhaps because no software was available. Usually, the statistician discussed the protocol, helped in defining how data would be collected, and then disappeared or was ignored, until the last patient had been entered in the trial and was treated, or even until the last response had been obtained; this should no longer be the case.

On the contrary, early comparisons of the treatments can be the subject of controversies. Sequential analysis will not be discussed here. It is a solution to some of the difficulties discussed below, but its use is limited.

Arguments in favor of early comparisons are:

1. Concern about toxicity and side effects of one or several of the compared treatments. It is necessary to keep a close watch on the trial in order to stop it early if some striking results are observed.
2. Curiosity: since one expects the clinicians involved in the trial to be interested in the on-going comparison, it can be inferred that they are waiting impatiently for some results. It usually takes a long time to plan and initiate a trial; when it is underway at last, early results are expected. If the participating clinicians are not curious, interim analysis may stimulate their interest and participation.
3. The clinicians' impression that they have gathered enough evidence in favor of one of the treatments and need to support this impression by a statistical analysis.
4. The necessity to make a decision about the treatment of incoming patients, at the end of the accrual period, on the basis of the available data.
5. Publication of the results of another trial that studied one or several of the compared treatments.
6. Discovery of a new treatment that seems promising and seems to make the ongoing trial obsolete.

Arguments against early analysis are:

1. Repeated testing on accumulating data implies a greater risk of error than the risk used for each test.
2. The choice is difficult between decision and demonstration when a difference is observed which is interesting but not significant. On one hand, unconvincing results are produced; on the other hand, proceeding with the trial reluctantly may imply a bias in the selection of patients—such as removing from the trial a type of patient for which one treatment seemed better—or in the interpretation of the results.
3. Repeated analysis of survival rates creates special difficulties, since an improvement in short-term survival may be associated with a decline in long-term survival.

Is there a solution to the problem of interim analysis? Group sequential analysis[4] is certainly more practical for large trials than paired sequential analysis, but the problem of time lapse between patient entry and the observation of the response is just the same. For survival rates or any other time-related event several sequential solutions have been proposed for the analysis; for instance, sequential logrank test,[1] sequential Wilcoxon test, or Canner's test on hazard rates.[3]

Another solution is to compute the true significance level corresponding to n repeated tests at a given level.[2] This corresponds to the most current practice, although it has not been given much attention. It solves the statistical problem of the limitation of the risks of error, but not all the problems discussed here. Analysis of a trial is like an iceberg: the visible part, which is the published part, is very small as compared to the invisible part, all the interim analyses that are never published or even mentioned when the final results are published. Should the number of interim comparisons be given when the results of a trial are published? Or should the reader be left to wonder about the true level of significance, correcting the published data by guessing at the number of interim comparisons?

REFERENCES

1. Armitage, P. (1975). *Sequential Medical Trials*, 2nd ed., Blackwell Scientific Publications, Oxford.
2. Armitage, P.; McPherson, C. K., and Rowe, B. C. (1969) Repeated significance tests on accumulating data. *JR Statistic Soc*, **A132**: 235–44.
3. Canner, P. L., (1977). Monitoring treatment differences in long-term clinical trials. *Biometrics*,
4. Pocock, S. J. (1977). Group sequential methods in the design and analysis of clinical trials. *Biometrics* **64:** 2, 191–99.
5. Pocock, S. J., Armitage, P., and Galton, D. A. G. (1978). The size of cancer clinical trials: an international survey. *UICC Technical Report Series*, Vol. 36, pp. 5–34.

8

Feedback of Data to Participants During Clinical Trials

R. J. Prescott

Medical Computing and Statistics Unit, Medical School,
Edinburgh, Great Britain

CLINICAL TRIALS IN CANCER pose a number of problems for the statistician, both theoretical and practical, that are not encountered in applications outside medicine, nor indeed in many other areas of medicine. The particular topic covered in this chapter is certainly of this type. The question considered is what information about the data accumulated during progress of the trial should the trial statistician release to the other participants in the trial. In the course of discussing this question it will be argued that the trial statistician should accept much of the ethical responsibility in determining whether a trial should be allowed to continue.

The need to consider feedback of information to the participants in a cancer trial has its origin in the difficulty of obtaining adequate sample sizes for the trial. This requirement leads to many of the trials being multicentered, with entry of patients into the trial being spread over a considerable length of time.

The multicenter aspect almost certainly means that the motivation to undertake the extra work involved in participating in clinical trials will vary from unit to unit. Typically we might expect great enthusiasm from the originators of the trial, while those centers involved in a more peripheral way may be less strongly motivated. Furthermore, with entry of the patients into the trial extending over a lengthy period, perhaps several years, it may be difficult to maintain the initial motivation. Thus, there is a very real danger that the number of patients being entered into the trial will suffer a fall-off with time.

We can illustrate this phenomenon with data from a clinical trial concerning methods of treating early breast cancer. This trial was carried out in southeast Scotland, with patient entry between April, 1964 and March, 1971. The trial administration was centered in Edinburgh and will be referred to subsequently as the "Old Edinburgh Breast Trial." Women, aged 35–69, with clinical stage I or stage II disease and women with stage III disease, purely

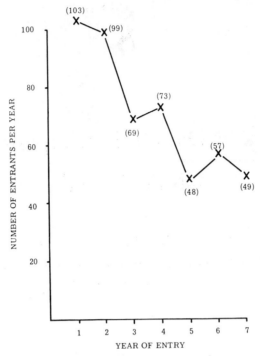

Fig. 1. Case entry to Edinburgh Breast Trial, 1964–71.

on account of size of tumor, were eligible for the trial. The treatments being compared were radical mastectomy and simple mastectomy plus radiotherapy. More details of the trial are given by Hamilton, Langlands, and Prescott.[2]

The number of patients entering the Old Edinburgh Breast Trial annually is shown in Figure 1. Entry was sustained at a high level for only two years before there was an appreciable drop in the admission rate.

This trial was undertaken with virtually no feedback to the participating surgeons responsible for entering patients, to let them know how the trial was progressing. As such, it represents one of the two possible extremes of policy with respect to feedback. Some possible unwanted side effects of this policy are

1. a gradual loss of identification with the aims of the study
2. new junior hospital staff may be inadequately instructed in trial procedures
3. deviations from the trial protocol are more likely
4. participants become more easily influenced by reports in the literature of alternative treatments or become prejudiced in favor of one of the alternatives used in the trial.

These factors work to bring about not only a fall-off in the number of patients admitted to the study but, perhaps as important, tend to reduce the quality of information recorded on those admitted to the study.

The policy of no feedback undoubtedly owes a great deal to the dangers of giving too much information to participants while the trial is progressing:

1. *Repeated significance tests:* It is well recognized that the repeated application of fixed-sample-size tests of significance destroys the usual interpretation of any significance level reported. In presenting the application of repeated significance tests as a danger when feedback is detailed, there is no suggestion that the trial statistician would draw unsound inferences. However, some participants may be tempted to see "how significant" the results are to date, and if application of an appropriate (or indeed inappropriate) fixed-sample-size test yields $p < 0.05$, the trial statistician may be placed in a very difficult position. However cogently he argues that the observed significance level is invalid he will meet the other main problem.

2. *Ethical problems for the participants:* The above example illustrates the dilemma that a doctor may experience when he has detailed knowledge of how the trial results are progressing. Viewed objectively he may accept the statistician's argument. Taking a dispassionate view, he may reason that it is worth increasing the risk for some patients in the short term in order to obtain information that will bring benefit to the long-term patient population. However, faced with the next patient who is a potential entrant for the trial he must take a very difficult decision. Undoubtedly, many doctors will decide that it is unethical to continue the trial in such circumstances.

This example is extreme, but it will be common at some stage in most trials for the survival curves to show visually different survivals for the two groups. This may not approach conventional levels of significance, even for a fixed-sample-size test, but nevertheless will be sufficient to raise ethical difficulties for the participants.

If the trial is stopped prematurely because of ethical concern from the participants, this may (though may not) be beneficial to potential trial entrants. However, it will lessen the confidence of doctors outside the trial in any published results of the trial. It is not farfetched to suggest that it may stop or delay the widespread application of a beneficial treatment.

An early end to the trial will also pose a problem in statistical inference for the trial statistician. In practice, the results will have been examined sequentially and a fixed-sample-size analysis would be difficult to justify. However, how can the sequential element be handled under such an ill-defined stopping rule?

Thus there is a clear pointer to the need for a policy of feedback of information somewhere between the two extremes of giving no information and giving detailed results. Such an intermediate policy was implemented in a subsequent study of breast cancer in women aged less than 70, carried out in southeast Scotland between April, 1974 and March, 1978. We will refer to this study as the "New Edinburgh Breast Trial." The range of patients eligible for this study was slightly wider than for the Old Edinburgh Breast Trial (Duncan et al.)[1], and so a direct comparison of numbers entered is inappropriate. The study comprised two trials. In trial I, patients with clinical stage I or II with no histological evidence of pectoral node involvement were treated either by simple mastectomy and immediate postoperative radiotherapy or by simple mastectomy alone with radiotherapy delayed until evidence of local recurrence was apparent. Trial II was to assess the effect of adjuvant chemotherapy. Patients were those with stage I or II disease with histological evidence of pectoral node involvement and patients with stage III disease, operable or inoperable. The standard treatment alone (radiotherapy and, if operable, simple mastectomy) was compared with the standard treatment plus chemotherapy using 5-fluorouracil.

TABLE I
Intake for First 3½ Years of Breast Trials[a]

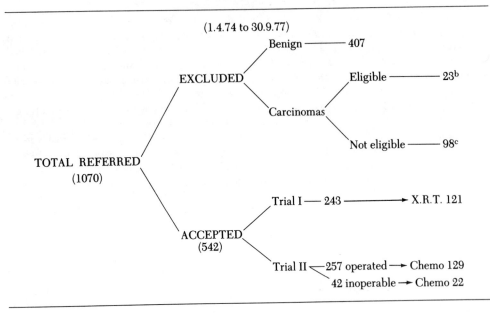

(1.4.74 to 30.9.77)

Benign ———— 407

EXCLUDED

Carcinomas

Eligible ———— 23[b]

Not eligible ———— 98[c]

TOTAL REFERRED
(1070)

Trial I — 243 ————→ X.R.T. 121

ACCEPTED
(542)

Trial II ⟨ 257 operated —→ Chemo 129
42 inoperable —→ Chemo 22

[a] April 1, 1974 to September 30, 1977
[b,c] The trial report gives a further breakdown of these cases.

For these trials it was arranged in advance that an annual report would be sent to participants, but in practice half-yearly reports were distributed. The trial committee agreed that information on treatment differences would not be released by the statistician during the accrual of patients. To avoid any ethical problems that this would pose, the results would be examined annually and entry to the trial stopped if differences in survival (on a fixed-sample-size test) were significant at the 0.1% level. With this strategy, the observed significance levels from fixed-sample-size tests applied at the normal completion of the trial would be little affected by the intermediate analysis. We note that this approach is broadly similar to that advocated by Peto[3] for use of the sequential logrank test.

As any reference to the effect of treatment was to be omitted from the reports the data presented had of necessity to be fairly basic and limited. The format for the results was not identical for all reports, in the hope that this would make them more interesting to their audience. Certain basic information was always given. This included a breakdown of the number of referrals to the trial (Table I). Another rather complicated table was also presented regularly (Table II). Two features of this table are important. First, it conveys information on what is happening in the trial within the wider context of breast cancer in the region. Second, it presents this information serially, so that the participants can see that the momentum of the trial is being maintained.

Additional tables presented were chosen either because of their potential interest to the participants or in order to draw attention to important features of the trial protocol. Thus Table III implicitly reminds the participants of the importance of obtaining a pectoral node

TABLE II
Cases of Breast Carcinoma Referred to Radiotherapy Department[a]

	Totals	Half-yearly						
		1st	2nd	3rd	4th	5th	6th	7th
Inclusions in trials								
1. Eligible, referred, accepted	542	72	78	60	60	103	86	83
2. Eligible, referred, accepted, withdrawn	23	7	3	1	7	1	3	1
Exclusions—Eligible Cases								
3. Eligible but referred postoperatively	92	15	11	14	10	10	18	14
4. Eligible but not referred (participating surgeons)	83	20	14	15	11	9	10	4
Subtotal	740	114	106	90	88	123	117	102
% Referred	76	69	76	68	76	85	76	82
5. Eligible but not referred (nonparticipating surgeons)	270	42	45	39	41	36	32	35
Exclusions—Ineligible Cases								
6. Referred	87	8	11	12	13	12	12	19
7. Not referred	440[b]	64	71	68	57	49	80	51
Grand total	1537	228	233	209	199	220	241	207

[a] From April, 1, 1974 to September 30, 1977 (3½ years).
[b] 308 > 70 years of age

TABLE III
Rates of Failure of Node Sampling[a]

	Numbers with no node histology/number treated (%)		
	Clinical stage I	Clinical stage II	Total
Consultant surgeon	50/152 (33%)	18/99 (18%)	68/251 (27%)
Trainee surgeon	29/63 (46%)	12/47 (26%)	41/110 (37%)
Totals	79/215 (37%)	30/146 (21%)	109/361 (30%)

[a] In 361 trial patients with clinical stages I and II breast cancer.

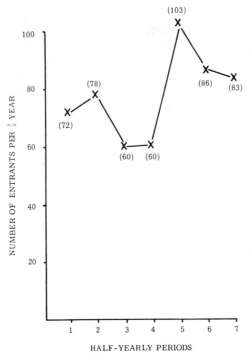

Fig. 2.   Case entry to New Edinburgh Breast Trial, 1974–77.

for histological examination and draws attention to the relative lack of success of junior surgeons in obtaining these nodes. A possibly important administrative point about the production of these tables and the half-yearly report is that the trial doctor, rather than the statistician, suggested the content, and the trial committee worked from this draft. Intuitively it seems plausible that the study doctor will be more aware of what features will seem relevant to medical colleagues. Indeed, to the statistician, the information available for feedback, excluding as it does any data on the outcome of treatment, may all seem extremely dull.

The real test on whether interest in the trial is maintained is provided by the entry of patients into the trial. In this case, entry to the trial was maintained at a high level throughout the first three-and-a-half years of the trial for which data are currently available (Figure 2).

Although the data presented in this paper on intake into the Edinburgh breast trials are too limited to draw sweeping conclusions, they are suggestive that feedback of information may help in maintaining the interest of participants in the trial. The New Edinburgh Breast Trial certainly establishes that it is possible to maintain a high rate of entry into a multi-centered clinical trial over an extended period of time.

As important as the question of what information should be circulated to participants is the question of what information should be restricted to the trial statistician alone. The statistician should be fully aware that by releasing any information about the outcome of patients in the trial he is placing what might prove to be an intolerable ethical burden on his medical colleagues. Equally, in withholding information he must ensure that the conduct of the trial is seen to safeguard the interests of the trial patients. This can only point to the data being tested sequentially. Clearly any decision on the release or nonrelease of information and the sequential analysis can only be made with the agreement of all parties. In keeping the outcome confidential the statistician is of course taking the bulk of the ethical responsibility on his own shoulders, but in the cancer-trial situation, the statistician is perhaps the best-placed person to do so.

REFERENCES

1. Duncan, W.; Langlands, A. O.; Forrest, A. P. M.; Prescott, R. J.; Gray, N.; Shivas, A. A.; Hamilton, T.; and Stewart, H. J. (1975). New Edinburgh Primary Breast Cancer Trials. *Br J Cancer*, **32**: 628–30.
2. Hamilton, T.; Langlands, A. O.; and Prescott, R. J. (1974). The treatment of operable cancer of the breast: a clinical trial in the South-east Region of Scotland. *Br J Surg*, **61**: 758–61.
3. Peto, R. (1978). This volume.

Can Sequential Methods be Used for the Analysis of Cancer Clinical Trials?

Stuart J. Pocock

Department of Clinical Epidemiology and Social Medicine
Royal Free Hospital, Pond Street
London NW3
England

1. INTRODUCTION

IN THE EXECUTION OF ANY CLINICAL TRIAL for the treatment of cancer it is generally considered unethical and also very inefficient to wait until the results on all patients have been obtained before making any inferences about the effectiveness of treatments. In statistical parlance the "fixed sample size" approach is unacceptable. Nevertheless many trial protocols specify a fixed number of patients, often with certain statistical design objectives in mind, but one assumes from experience that the trial organizers do not intend to be as inflexible as they imply.

At the other extreme there exist methods of sequential design and analysis geared to the idea that after every additional patient on each treatment has been evaluated, some formal statistical stopping rules are applied to determine whether the whole trial should stop or continue. Such a sequential approach involves certain assumptions:

1. the response variable conforms to some standard statistical distribution
2. patients enter in matched pairs (one to each treatment)
3. patient evaluation is instantaneous
4. constant surveillance is made of the accumulating data

The situation for a typical cancer clinical trial is rather different:

1. response is measured either by tumor shrinkage, disease-free interval, or patient survival, each of which take months or years to observe

2. patients vary with respect to several prognostic factors, and, although stratification can be a partial solution, pairing of patients is impractical
3. patient entry from several hospitals will require a complex system of central data collection, which entails some delay between patient evaluation at the hospital and inclusion of his outcome in the analysis
4. the statistician and trial organizers will normally be too busy to maintain a constant vigil over the data in order to observe the point at which a sequential boundary is crossed.

There is a sharp contrast between the theoretical ideal of sequential methods and the practical situation of cancer clinical trials, so that the simple answer to the question posed by the title of this paper is NO! This is certainly my own experience, since I am unaware of any cancer clinical trial that has successfully implemented a sequential design.

So neither fixed sample size nor conventional sequential methods are applicable. Instead the cancer clinical trial will normally proceed with some inspection of results from time to time with an informal interpretation by the trial organizers as to whether any action to stop or change a treatment is justified. Some fixed sample size significance tests may be used to aid decision making, but the overall approach is subjective. One might take the defeatist standpoint that *any* more formalized approach to the design and analysis of trials is unrealistic. However, I think this is liable to result in a very unscientific approach to clinical trials, whereby the statistical validity of conclusions remains uncertain.

What is needed is a method of statistical design and analysis that takes into account the fact that it is common practice to assess the accumulating results of an ongoing trial at several equally spaced time points, each of which might normally occur prior to a meeting of the trial organizers. This paper describes one such general type of *group sequential* design based on the repeated use of conventional significance testing.

However, before we go into the details of such an approach, it is as well to consider the current status of clinical trial practice.

2. A SURVEY ON THE SIZE OF CANCER TRIALS

This survey was undertaken for the UICC Project on Controlled Therapeutic Trials by Pocock, Armitage, and Galton.[6] The main objectives of the survey are to find out:

1. Do investigators determine the required size of trial in advance?
2. How successful are they in accruing an adequate number of patients?
3. Do they assess interim results while the trial is in progress and do such analyses affect the eventual size of trial?

The sampling frame for the survey was the 334 trials registered with the UICC information office from 1972 to mid-1975. A random sample of 50 trials was chosen and a questionnaire sent to each principal investigator. Replies were received from 40 (80%), and the responses to the most relevant questions are presented in below in three sections:

a. Design
In 34/40 cases (85%) the required number of patients was specified before the trial began.

The actual number was recorded in 26 cases and the distribution was as follows:

9 trials required	45–90	patients (all treatments combined)			
12 " "	100–200	"	"	"	"
1 " "	210	"	"	"	"
1 " "	400+	"	"	"	"
2 " "	500	"	"	"	"
1 " "	1690	"	"	"	"

The methods of determining the required sample size were as follows:

18 used power calculations for a fixed number of patients
8 made a subjective decision, without statistical methods
1 used a sequential design, which was abandoned later
3 made somewhat unusual statistical statements
4 used statistical methods, with no details given

Thus, statistical power calculations for determining a fixed size of trial seem the most popular approach. This involves:

1. making a decision as to what is the smallest difference in treatment effects that it is important to detect
2. defining a single significance test and level (say $P < .05$) to be used once only at the end of the trial as the criterion for detecting that a difference exists and
3. specifying a degree of certainty (say 90%) that the detection method 2 for the underlying difference 1 would be successful. The required number of patients can thence be obtained from a simple statistical formula.

This method can give rise to a very wide range of sample size needs as illustrated in this survey. The 1,690 patients required in one trial reflects a statistician's excessive adherence to this approach without consideration of what was a feasible rate of accruing patients. A more realistic approach is normally adopted, whereby the power calculations are made to fit in with a preliminary subjective decision based on how long a trial should last and the availability of suitable patients. Thus, the statistical methods are used as a check on the scientific acceptability of a choice already made on practical grounds. This seems reasonable provided the statistical statements 1–3 above do not become too optimistic. Unfortunately, in eight of the above trials a 100% difference in median survival or median disease-free interval was used as the basis for power calculations, which resulted in relatively small sample size requirements of around 30–50 patients per treatment. This enthusiasm of investigators for small phase III trials in the hope of very large treatment differences is a considerable hindrance to progress in cancer research.

b. Realization

At the time of this survey only half of the trials had terminated patient accrual, so that one cannot give an overall picture of their eventual outcome. However, since all trials had been in progress for at least two years, one can study the mean annual accrual rates. This information was available for 39 trials and the distribution is as follows:

3 trials entered	<10	patients per annum			
8 "	"	10–19	"	"	"
6 "	"	20–29	"	"	"
8 "	"	30–49	"	"	"
8 "	"	50–79	"	"	"
5 "	"	100–199	"	"	"
		266			

Another way of considering a trial's progress is to calculate the number of years of patient accrual required to achieve the target number specified in the trial's design. This information was available for 24 trials and the distribution is as follows:

No. trials	Years required
3	<2
2	2–3
7	3–4
7	4–8
5	>10

In summary, the median accrual rate is 33 patients per annum, and the median time to achieve the specified accrual target is over four years. Clearly, this is a very unsatisfactory situation, which results in many trials either failing to achieve adequate patient numbers or becoming excessively protracted. Further study of the survey results indicates that both single institution and multicenter trials experience these problems. Until all trial organizers obtain a truly realistic assessment of the potential patient accrual and ensure the full co-operation of all contributing investigators, the problem of poor accrual will continue to ruin a large proportion of clinical trials.

c. Analysis

Investigators were asked whether they had undertaken any form of *interim* or *ongoing analysis* of results while the trial was in progress. 33/40 (83%) responded Yes, and the frequency of interim analysis was as follows:

Every three months	1
Every four months	9
Every six months	13
Every year	3
Every two years or less	2
Sequential analysis	2
One toxicity analysis only	2
Unknown	1

Evaluation of trial every four to six months seems a very common practice, which is probably linked to the tri- or biannual meetings of the trial organizers. One of the two sequential analyses was eventually abandoned, while the other involved a separate sequential treatment comparison within each of several patient strata with reporting of results every 3 months, so that neither remained truly sequential. Six of the seven who had not undertaken interim analyses implied they would do so once there was sufficient data.

Investigators were also asked whether they used any formal or informal *stopping rules* regarding the early termination of trial if treatment differences should develop. The 38 replies were as follows:

22 had no stopping rules
 2 used sequential methods, as mentioned earlier
 6 used repeated significance testing
 4 adopted a subjective approach based on the magnitude of treatment difference
 1 used a peculiar statistical argument
 3 used some stopping rule, but gave no details

Thus the majority had no agreed policy as to early termination of trial. This is unfortunate, since the whole objective is to identify a superior treatment and to ensure that patients will not receive an inferior treatment once a difference is clearly established.

Repeated significance testing means that at periodic intervals, say every six months, one or more significance tests are carried out to see if there is evidence of a treatment difference. If statistical significance is reached at some point, this will be used as the basis for a decision to stop the trial. This approach seems quite sensible in that, unlike many sequential designs, it is readily understood by both statisticians and clinicians. However, there are three major problems which need to be clarified:

1. If there are several measures of a patient's response to treatment, e.g., tumor shrinkage, survival, toxicity, disease-free interval, then it is quite likely that some will show significant differences and others will not. This presents a logical problem, which may be overcome by giving primary importance to one variable and using other comparisons as a more informal check that the superiority of one treatment follows a consistent pattern. Alternatively, one could define some single more complex multivariate significance test based on all relevant variables, but this may be unrealistic in the case of such disparate factors as tumor response and toxicity.

2. Clinical investigators cannot be expected to accept a significance test as the sole criterion for stopping a trial. Previous experience, evidence from trials in other centers, and the degree of enthusiasm for the trial will all necessarily be taken into account. Thus the ultimate decision will be a subjective one, but it is important that statistical evidence be a primary factor.

3. The more often a significance test is performed on the accumulating results in a trial, the greater is the chance that some significant difference will eventually be detected, even if the treatments are really equally effective. This fact will tend to contribute to an excess of false positive results reported in the clinical trial literature. Hence repeated examination of data means that one must set a more stringent significance level than $P < .05$, and this

point is discussed further in the next section. However, before we approach this more statistical topic it may be helpful to state the following simple rule:

If one expects to take up to a maximum of 10 repeated looks at the data during the course of a trial, then a significance level of $P < 0.01$ should be adopted as the criterion for stopping the trial, since the chance of drawing a *false* conclusion that one treatment is superior is roughly equivalent to making a decision based on a single test at the level $P < 0.05$.

3. GROUP SEQUENTIAL ANALYSIS

This section describes how repeated significance testing of accumulating data can be formulated as a precise method of statistical analysis for clinical trials. Armitage[1] describes several RST sequential designs based on significance testing after each pair of patients, one to each treatment. However, as mentioned in Section 1, this continual testing has both theoretical and practical difficulties. Instead we consider the *group sequential* approach, whereby significance tests are performed at longer equally spaced intervals. The results and methods described here are based on Pocock,[5] and further reference to the same general approach can be obtained from McPherson.[3,4]

First, we return to the problem that repeated significance tests increase the *overall significance level*, that is, the probability of at least one significant difference when the treatments are really the same. Table I shows the results for repeated two-sided testing at the 5% level at equally spaced numbers of patients with two treatments and a normally distributed response variable with constant known variance, though broadly similar results hold for any type of response variable and any pattern of repeated testing. For only 10 re-

TABLE I
Repeated Significance Tests on Accumulating Data[a]

No. of repeated significance tests at the 5% level	Overall significance level
1	0.05
2	0.08
3	0.11
4	0.13
5	0.14
10	0.19
20	0.25
50	0.32
100	0.37
1,000	0.53
∞	1

[a] Two treatments and a normal response variable.

peated tests the overall significance level has increased from 0.05 to 0.19, and with more and more repeated testing one can become increasingly sure that a treatment difference will be declared whether one is really present or not. Clearly the naive application of repeated significance testing allows the unscrupulous investigator ample scope to demonstrate some significant advance in the treatment of cancer!

The way to correct for this problem is to choose a lower, more stringent *nominal significance level* for each repeated test, so that the overall significance level is 0.05. Table II shows what these nominal levels need to be for the case of a normal response, though simulation has shown that the same nominal levels are accurate for a wide variety of response variables. Furthermore, these results hold for more elaborate tests involving adjustment for covariates and are not sensitive to variations away from exactly equal numbers of additional patients between tests.

This simple adjustment can thus make repeated significance testing a respectable statistical tool, the only restriction being that one must decide in advance how many repeated tests are to be performed.

Let us illustrate the approach with data from an actual trial of two drug combinations, CP (cytoxan-prednisone) and CVP (cytoxan-vincristine-prednisone), for the treatment of advanced non-Hodgkins lymphoma. The main criterion for response was tumor shrinkage, and Figure 1 shows how the response rates on the two treatments varied over the course of the trial, with patient accrual from June, 1972 to October, 1974. It can be seen that every time a patient is evaluated the response rate changes, and, as in the early stages of any trial, this leads to wild fluctuations. However, as patient numbers increase, the curves inevitably become more stable.

Now, suppose the intention was to have about 120–130 patients on the trial and to analyze the accumulating data on five occasions; that is, after about every 25 patients. This would lead to analyses at the times marked ↑ in Figure 1 with the following results:

		Response Rates			
		CP	CVP	χ^2 (without continuity correction)	
January	1973	3/14	5/11	1.63	
July	1973	11/27	13/24	0.92	
November	1973	18/40	17/36	0.04	
April	1974	18/54	24/47	3.25	$0.05 < P < 0.1$
October	1974	23/67	31/59	4.25	Nominal Significance Level $< P < .05$

At each of the five time points the response rates are compared using a χ^2 test without continuity correction, with the intention of stopping the trial if $P < 0.0158$, the nominal significance level obtained from Table II. The lack of continuity correction is necessary so that the repeated testing is not unduly conservative; see Pocock.[5] Even with $P < 0.05$ on the final test a treatment difference could not be declared significant at the 5% level, since the nominal P-value of 0.0158 was not achieved. Of course, it would not be desirable

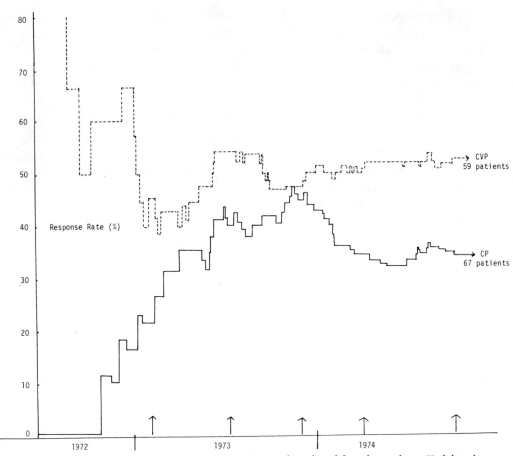

Fig. 1. Cumulative response rates for two treatments in a clinical trial for advanced non-Hodgkins lymphoma

TABLE II
Nominal Significance Levels[a]

No. of repeated significance tests	Nominal significance level
2	0.0294
3	0.0221
4	0.0182
5	0.0158
10	0.0106
15	0.0086
20	0.0075

[a] Corresponding to an overall significance level of 0.05 (normal response).

to take a totally negative interpretation for this trial. In practice one would infer from this data alone that the superiority of CVP with regard to tumor response is interesting but inconclusive. Eventually, further data on the duration of response and patient survival would help to clarify the situation.

Superficially, this example illustrates the ease with which group sequential methods can be used. In fact, there are several difficulties which my conscience compels me to raise. Tumor response is not observed instantaneously and can take up to several weeks to observe. The simplest solution is to allow a fixed period, say three months, to observe whether response occurs in a patient. This means that analysis after each group of patients takes place three months later than was indicated above, i.e., the first analysis would have been April 1973, not January 1973. Such an unavoidable delay means that further patients will have entered the trial in the interim, and this may raise complications if the nominal significance level is achieved and the trial is stopped. If stopping the trial means that all patients still receiving the inferior treatment are taken off it instantaneously, then there will be no further direct data on response and the treatment comparison remains unaltered. However, if it is thought appropriate for patients entered but not evaluated to complete their current therapy, then there will be further response data, which may slightly alter the final treatment comparison. This can lead to contradictions if the results become less significant, but should not be a serious problem unless the delay to observe response is unduly long.

In this regard there may be administrative delay in getting the observed response reported for inclusion in analysis. In multicenter cooperative groups this can be a matter of months, in which case any stopping rule becomes hopelessly delayed. For instance, the above example illustrates the preferred way of conducting the ongoing analysis of the trial, whereas in practice the delays were such that the final response data were not analyzed until over a year after the last patient was entered. It seems to me that for the benefit of patients participating in clinical trials there must be a considerable improvement in the feedback and processing of response data in order that a prompt analysis can be carried out and any inferior treatment detected.

4. GROUP SEQUENTIAL DESIGNS

We now consider how the method of repeated significance testing can be formulated into the design of a clinical trial, particularly as regards power calculations. The two features to be decided on at the start of such a group sequential trial are:

1. How many significance tests should there be—that is, what is the maximum number of groups?
2. How many patients should be evaluated before each significance test—that is, what should be the size of each group?

Let us here consider a trial with two treatments, $2n$ patients per group (n per treatment) and a maximum of N groups. This makes the maximum size of trial = $2nN$ patients.

The method of determining the operating characteristics of designs with a variety of values for n and N is described in Pocock.[5] Here we consider the simplest theoretical case

TABLE III
Group Sequential Designs for a Normal Response[a]

Maximum no. of groups (N)	Required no. of patients per group (2n)	Maximum no. of patients (2nN)	Average no. of patients to termination of trial under H_A
1	42.04	42.04	42.04
2	23.12	46.24	32.60
3	16.11	48.33	30.29
4	12.43 $\times \dfrac{\sigma^2}{\delta^2}$	49.72 $\times \dfrac{\sigma^2}{\delta^2}$	29.33 $\times \dfrac{\sigma^2}{\delta^2}$
5	10.14	50.70	28.80
10	5.35	53.50	28.03
20	2.79	55.80	27.98

[a] With known variance σ^2, overall significance level $\alpha = 0.05$, and power $1 - \beta = 0.09$ under H_A: $\mu_A - \mu_B = \delta$.

of two treatment groups, for each of which we have a normally distributed response with means μ_A, μ_B and known variance σ^2. The conventional power calculation here requires specification of an overall significance level α and power $1 - \beta$ for a specific alternative hypothesis $\mu_A - \mu_B = \delta$. Tables derived by numerical integration enable the required value of n for any given N to be determined, but for limitations of space let us here just consider the results for $\alpha = 0.05$ and $1 - \beta = 0.9$ that are presented in Table III. Remember that the required nominal significance levels for any choice of N are to be found in Table II. Clearly, as the number of groups N increases, the number per group $2n$ decreases and the maximum number of patients $2nN$ increases. However, the most important feature in a group sequential design is the extent to which it enables early termination of trial when the alternative hypothesis is true. This is indicated in the last column of Table III by the average sample size. Evidently the greatest reduction is achieved by using a two-group design instead of a one-group (i.e., fixed sample size) design, and there appears little advantage in using a design with more than five groups. This applies to any trial design based on $\alpha = 0.05$ and $\beta = 0.9$, and similar examples could be evaluated for other values of α and β. The only advantage of designs with a large number of groups (i.e., repeated significance tests) is in the very early detection of extremely large treatment differences. Consider one extreme case of repeated significance testing after every pair of patients (i.e., an RST sequential design) for $\alpha = 0.05$, $1 - \beta = 0.9$ and $\delta = 0.5 \sigma$. The required maximum sample size is 242 and the average sample size under H_A is 116.6 compared with 115.2 for the equivalent five-group design. Thus, continual significance testing is an actual handicap compared with occasional testing at five equally spaced intervals.

Of course the response variable in a clinical trial rarely follows a normal distribution, but for trials with relatively few groups this is not a serious problem, since asymptotic normal approximations can be used with sufficient accuracy. In particular, Pocock[5] describes how binary and exponential responses can be used for group sequential designs. Also, in most trials it is important to allow for prognostic factors in making treatment comparisons, but, provided one does not include too many factors, the inclusion of covariate adjustment in analysis will have no serious effect on the operation characteristics of group sequential designs.

5. SURVIVAL DATA

It is becoming widely accepted that most survival data are best analyzed by nonparametric methods. Armitage[1] and Jones and Whitehead[2] have considered sequential analysis based on the logrank test. However, repeated analysis after every death would be an exhausting exercise, and instead I wish to consider here how a group sequential approach could be used.

The usual group sequential testing described in Sections 3 and 4 is at equally spaced numbers of patients, whereas for the logrank test it would seem more appropriate, and asymptotically equivalent, to analyze at *equally spaced numbers of deaths*. The theoretical details have not been worked out as yet, but I believe that the nominal significance levels in Table II would provide an overall significance level of 0.05 for a logrank group sequential design. Further research would also be needed to define power calculations in this context.

Such an approach would mean that a considerable time would elapse between the start of the trial and the first analysis, but the time intervals between analyses would then shorten as more patients were entered and deaths occurred more frequently. In this way any unduly premature survival analyses based on very few deaths would be avoided.

The success of group sequential survival designs depends primarily on the speed with which deaths are reported. The consequences of an early significant result may be just the cessation of patient entry, but if treatment is ongoing (e.g., long-term chemotherapy), use of the inferior treatment on patients already entered may also cease, so that the whole trial is closed. In this latter case, there will be no further data to add to the survival comparison except as a result of administrative delay, but in the former case there will be greater difficulty of statistical interpretation as further survival follow-up continues. This problem of a stopping rule being followed by further data has not been satisfactorily resolved, but the best approach may be a conventional fixed-sample-size analysis of the final data with some informal acknowledgement that a stopping rule has been used.

6. SECRECY OF INTERIM ANALYSES

Repeated presentation of interim results can have considerable influence on the participating investigators. An early interim analysis showing treatment comparisons can have disastrous effects on the future progress of a trial. If there is little difference between treatments some investigators may lose interest. However, a more serious situation arises if there are interesting differences which are not statistically significant. Some participants may then drop out of the trial, arguing that they believe there is a genuine difference, while others may continue in a half-hearted manner with perhaps an increased tendency to adapt the supposedly inferior treatment, remove patients from it prematurely or, worse still, interfere with the randomization.

Investigators may not be happy with complete secrecy, so a compromise solution may be required whereby results are presented for all treatments, combined with an additional statement that there is no significant difference as yet. Some small committee, perhaps made up of one statistician and a nonparticipating clinician, could keep a detailed check on the interim results, which would only be presented to others in full when treatment differences are of sufficient magnitude to merit termination of the trial.

An additional problem is the premature publication of results while a trial is still in progress, which has the more serious effect that the whole medical community may be prejudiced towards a particular conclusion before the full results are known. Such early public presentation took place in at least 7 of the 40 trials surveyed in Section 2.

CONCLUSIONS

1. For most clinical trials in cancer some form of informal ongoing analysis of results is undertaken, though conventional sequential methods are hardly ever used.
2. This practice of periodically analyzing the accumulating data can be formulated more precisely as a group sequential design whereby stopping rules are based on repeated significance testing at equal intervals. There appears no great advantage in carrying out many repeated tests, both for statistical reasons and because of the effort involved. One sensible design would be to plan for no more than ten repeated analyses, with a decision to stop the trial if the main treatment difference is significant at the 1% level.
3. Such statistical stopping rules can never be rigorously applied but should improve the objectivity of decision making.
4. Difficulties in obtaining adequate patient accrual, administrative inefficiency, and premature dissemination of results are major faults in the organization of many cancer trials, for which no amount of statistical refinement can correct.

REFERENCES

1. Armitage, P. (1975). *Sequential Medical Trials*, Blackwell, Oxford.
2. Jones, D. R., and Whitehead, J. (1978). Sequential forms of the logrank and modified wilcoxon tests for censored survival data. (In preparation.)
3. McPherson, K. (1974). Statistics: The problem of examining accumulating data more than once. *New Eng J Med* 290: 501–2.
4. McPherson, K. (1977). "Sequential Analysis of Clinical Trial Data." In *Clinical Trials*, F. N. and S. Johnson (Eds.), Blackwell, Oxford.
5. Pocock, S. J. (1977). Group sequential methods in the design and analysis of clinical trials. *Biometrika*, 64: 191–99.
6. Pocock, S. J.; Armitage, P.; and Galton, D. A. G. (1978). The size of cancer clinical trials: An international survey. Submitted to the *Int J Cancer*.

CHAPTER

10

The Necessity and Justification of Randomized Clinical Trials

David P. Byar

Clinical and Diagnostic Trials Section, Biometry Branch
National Cancer Institute, NIH
Bethesda, Maryland 20205
U.S.A.

ALTHOUGH I DID NOT personally choose the title of this presentation, I can certainly live with it because I do believe that randomized clinical trials are necessary. This does not mean that all studies of treatment in patients with cancer must be randomized clinical trials, but rather that there will always be situations in which randomized clinical trials will be necessary if we are to use the best means of judging treatment efficacy.

Dr. Ed Gehan, who is one of the statisticians who has spoken most consistently in favor of historically controlled studies, is engaged in organizing and analyzing many randomized clinical trials and has been doing so for many years. In a recent paper published in *Biomedicine*[1] as part of the proceedings of a conference held in Paris earlier this year concerned with precisely the problems which we are discussing today, Dr. Gehan points out, and I quote: "Randomized studies are useful when there is no basis for choosing comparable patients treated in the past, that is when patient characteristics related to prognosis are not well known." In addition he points out that "When studies may be expected to last five years or more, it is difficult to foresee all the changes that might take place, so it may be reasonable to do a randomized study."

It appears that this increasingly popular debate, pitting randomizers against nonrandomizers, is not a matter of principle but a matter of degree. Even I, who along with seven coauthors wrote a widely read paper (judging from the number of reprint requests) defending randomization[2], am often involved in analyzing data from nonrandomized studies. The important question to be considered in making this choice is what are the characteristics of situations in which nonrandomized trials might be reasonable and appropriate, and which are those that require a randomized study. This topic has been so vigorously debated over the last few years that I am beginning to feel more like an evangelist than a scientist when discussing it, involving as it does faith and judgment to perhaps a larger extent than logic and reason. By the end of May, 1978 there will have been five major meetings (two in Europe and three in the United States) in the past year concerned with the design of clinical trials. One might ask, why so much emphasis on methodology? Professor G. W. Pickering,[3] in his presidential address to the Royal Society of Medicine entitled "The Place of the Experimental Method in Medicine," answers this question by quoting Karl Pearson: "The true aim of the teacher should be to impart an appreciation of method and not a knowledge of facts," and goes on to comment that method is retained as an attitude of mind even when the facts have been forgotten. I must restrain myself from quoting further from this wise and delightfully written address.

PURPOSE OF CLINICAL TRIALS

Before comparing randomized clinical trials with studies based on historical control groups, we must first state the purpose of a comparative clinical trial. I will assume that the purposes of a clinical trial are: (1) to find out which (if any) of two or more treatments is more effective and (2) to convince other researchers of the results. I suspect that in the past too little attention has been paid to this second objective and I shall have more to say about that later.

HETEROGENEITY OF PATIENTS

With such simple objectives we may well inquire why we need statistics at all. The reason for this is clearly that patients are very heterogeneous and the course of most cancers is highly variable and influenced by many factors other than treatment. To illustrate this point I would like to describe a recent analysis of prognostic factors in thyroid cancer based on data collected by the EORTC thyroid registry. During preliminary analysis it was learned that prognosis for patients with thyroid cancer depended on a number of factors, including the patient's age, sex, histology of the tumor, the size and location of the tumor, and the extent of metastasis. By fitting a regression model based on the Weibull distribution to the survival times of thyroid cancer patients, we were able to divide the entire group of 507 patients into five risk groups (see Fig. 1). I find this a most startling picture because it demonstrates the extreme variability of this disease. It would be difficult to imagine separating the curves any further since they are almost touching the axes of the plot already! It should be apparent that any differences in survival attributable to different therapies are likely to be much smaller than those attributed to prognostic factors in this analysis. I have done similar analyses for patients with prostatic cancer and lung cancer, based on data collected from clinical trials of treatment of these two conditions. In both instances the separation of the curves by prognostic factors was markedly greater than that produced by the randomized treatments. This is one of the reasons that I am skeptical about the results of the historical

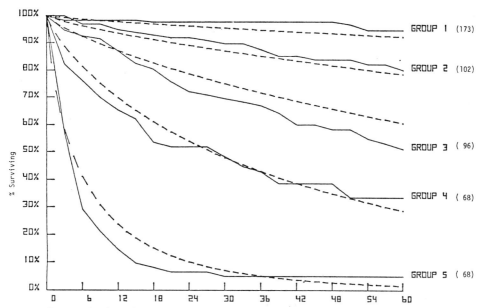

Fig. 1. Risk groups for thyroid cancer based on prognostic factors (see text). Solid lines represent actuarial curves, and dotted lines are predictions based on a Weibull survival model. Numbers of patients are shown in parentheses.

control studies. Admittedly it is possible to adjust to some extent for differences in base-line variables, but unfortunately we can only adjust for those variables we know about, and new ones are continually being discovered.

STUDIES WITH HISTORICAL CONTROLS

There are many reasons why studies relying on historical controls are considered to be desirable. The principal reasons usually cited are that fewer patients are required and thus the studies can be completed more quickly, that past information is efficiently used, that they are more ethical since all new patients are given the treatment for which there is greatest hope, and that they have worked well in the past. One cannot object to the claim that they take fewer patients or that they are completed more quickly. However, it is questionable how much faith should be placed in past information, and we are unable to support the claim that they have worked well in the past, since most of the therapeutic advances first discovered in historically controlled studies were later confirmed in randomized studies. We tend too easily to forget claims of therapeutic superiority which have not been reported elsewhere. The ethical argument is somewhat more complex. We may reasonably ask, if we do a study that convinces us but convinces no one else and is then either ignored or requires confirmation by yet another study, whether we have really acted in the most ethical fashion in the long run.

There are in addition some advantages of historically controlled studies that are usually not mentioned. One of these is that it is often possible to do a historically controlled study

TABLE I
Difficulties With Historical Controls

1. Absence of needed information for adjustment
2. Missing data
3. Reliance on mathematical assumptions
4. Possible time trends in:
   a. Patient population
   b. Diagnostic methods
   c. Details of treatment
   d. Supportive care
5. Effects of unmeasured or unknown prognostic factors
6. Failure to convince others of the results

at a single center. Thus we are not inconvenienced by the necessity of cooperation in a multicenter trial, nor are we likely to lose the personal credit that comes from principal or sole authorship of the published report. These, after all, are strong inducements to original scientific work and should not be ignored. In fact, some of the most innovative thinkers in medical therapeutics are those who do not favor randomized trials. They feel that their originality may be hampered by the inevitable compromises involved in mounting a multicenter randomized clinical trial. They would prefer to study 30 to 100 patients themselves, their personal series, and then move on to something else. I think that this is an unfortunate state of affairs since the results are often unsound, but the desire for personal recognition should not be taken as a criticism of randomized clinical trials. A better approach would be to find ways of integrating into the setting of randomized trials equitable methods for giving due scientific credit.

We may now turn to some arguments against the use of historical controls. These are listed in Table I. The first three items have to do with the necessity for performing adjusted comparisons. We may often find that information needed for adjustment is simply not available or is missing from many historical control patient's records. It would not be correct to use only patients for whom control information was available, since that might create systematic bias. In addition, all adjustment procedures rely on mathematical assumptions of one sort or another. These are often difficult to verify, and in any case adjustment procedures can never completely accomplish their objective. The fourth item on the list, possible time trends, is also difficult to evaluate but may definitely be quite important.

I should like to illustrate how the patient population may change in time. In a large study of treatment for prostatic cancer performed in the United States, patients were admitted over a period of eight years. In order to determine whether or not the patient population had changed during the study, I compared the survival experience of patients treated by placebo during the first $2\frac{1}{2}$ years of the study with those treated with estrogen during the last $2\frac{1}{2}$ years of the study. The difference was significant at $p < 0.01$. However, when I compared the two randomized treatments, either for all patients admitted to the study or just those admitted during the last $2\frac{1}{2}$ years, the difference was not significant. This seems clear evidence that the patient population changed in time.

I would also like to illustrate how changes in diagnostic methods can produce serious

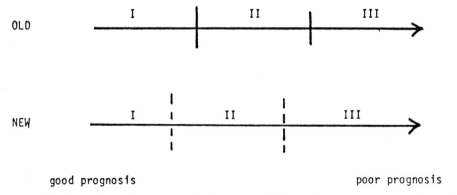

Fig. 2.   Possible effect of a new diagnostic method on staging which may bias treatment comparisons relying on historical controls. See text for explanation.

biases. In Figure 2, the two horizontal solid lines represent a continuum of a disease from good prognosis to bad prognosis. On the top line we imagine that, using old diagnostic methods, the disease can be conveniently divided into three stages labeled I, II, and III. For the lower line a new and more sensitive diagnostic method has been applied, allowing us to diagnose stage II and III patients at a somewhat earlier stage of the disease. If we imagine that patients on the top line represent historical controls and patients on the lower line represent those receiving a new treatment, it is clear that even in the absence of any superiority of the new treatment over that used for the historical controls, the change in diagnostic method would indicate improved survival in *all three stages*. There are fewer patients of poor prognosis in stages I and II and somewhat more patients with a better prognosis in stage III when we use the new diagnostic method.

The other two items listed under 4 in Table I, changes in the details of treatment or in general supportive care, may clearly affect the endpoints we wish to measure in a clinical trial. Generally, little information is available on these matters in historical records, and we are thus unable to measure their influence on our results. Item 5 has been mentioned above. It is clear that we cannot adjust for the effect of prognostic factors that are unknown to us or were never measured, yet we know that the effects of such factors may easily be greater than any possible treatment differences. Possibly the most serious difficulty with historical control studies is their failure to convince others of the results.

RANDOMIZED CLINICAL TRIALS

We may now turn to a discussion of randomized clinical trials. We usually use these terms to describe large multicenter trials, and such trials have recently been subject to sharp criticism. It has been argued that large multicenter trials suffer from a "dilution principle," a phrase intended to imply that the excellent results obtained in major centers are diluted by less striking results in other centers. I have been unable to find documentation that this principle is actually at work. Another recent idea is the "compromise principle," intended

TABLE II
Principal Advantages of Randomized Trials

1. Bias (conscious or unconscious) is avoided
2. Time trends are no problem, since they affect all treatment groups in the same way
3. Missing data are less likely, since all patients are following the same protocol
4. Mathematical models are not needed in the analysis
5. The results are more likely to be convincing
6. Randomized trials may be more ethical, since fewer patients need be treated to get a convincing answer

to describe a situation in which compromises concerning the nature or details of treatments must be reached in order for them to be acceptable to all centers involved in a large randomized trial. Again this charge is difficult to document and can only be considered a theoretical possibility. In fact, one might argue that the opinions of others are corrective and that a group of experts discussing possible treatments for cancer are more likely to arrive at reasonable ideas than single individuals who may be carried away by their own enthusiasm.

It is unquestionably true that there are many difficulties involved in running large-scale randomized trials, but I believe that the advantages of such studies, when well executed, clearly compensate for these difficulties. The principle advantages of randomized trials are given in Table II. An examination of this list reveals that randomized clinical trials may potentially correct many of the difficulties in historically controlled studies, and it is for this reason that their results are more likely to be convincing. Perhaps the greatest advantage of randomization is that it removes both conscious and unconscious bias from treatment assignment. This does not mean that the characteristics of patients in two treatment groups in a randomized trial will be identical. What it does mean is that a comparison of these two groups will be valid *despite* any imbalances, since the p-value obtained by applying a statistical test of significance takes into account the fact that such imbalances may occur. In fact, the p-value is a measure of just how probable a given difference in outcome would be in the absence of any real treatment differences. This does not mean, of course, that it may not be desirable to adjust for any differences in prognostic factors that may be observed, or to perform stratified analyses in order to increase the precision of treatment comparisons.

Problems with time trends in the nature of patients admitted to a study, changes in diagnostic procedures, or changes in general supportive care will not bias the results of a randomized trial, since such changes will affect all treatment groups to the same extent, provided that adaptive methods of treatment allocation are not used. This point has been discussed more fully in Byar et al.[2]

If a randomized trial is properly run, careful attention will have been given to exactly what data are to be recorded at entry to the study and at subsequent follow-up visits. These items should all be specified in the protocol with precise definitions to insure that the data are recorded uniformly for all patients. Those responsible for monitoring the study can see that all items are completed, and if some deficiencies are found, they can often be corrected during the course of the study. Such care is frequently not possible with historical records—we have to use what we find, hoping that the data are reasonably complete and that definitions have not changed too much. Unfortunately, we can never be sure to what extent our hopes are justified, and our conclusions must be tempered accordingly.

Even though it is often interesting and worthwhile to use mathematical models in analyzing the results of randomized trials, the principal conclusions relating to treatment comparisons do not depend on such analyses, and thus the usually unverifiable assumptions of such models need not affect our conclusions. Nonparametric methods of analysis, such as the logrank procedure discussed by Peto et al.,[4] are simple to understand and efficient from a statistical point of view.

ETHICAL PROBLEMS

Ethical problems can certainly arise in randomized trials, but it is illusory to think that they are absent in historically controlled studies. Ethics has to do with taking actions. Here the action is either to assign a patient to a particular therapy or to have the patient continue on that therapy. The problem arises when we think there is some evidence that one treatment may be better than another, a common problem as a trial progresses and begins to show promising signs in favor of one treatment or the other. One solution to this problem is to get all the patients into the trial as fast as possible before treatment results begin to emerge. We would still, of course, have the problem about whether to leave patients on what may appear to be an inferior therapy, but that concern will only apply if the treatment is one that is given continuously, such as a drug. It would not apply to an operation or a course of X-ray therapy. Even with a drug, it would be less clear from the results of the trial that patients still doing well on what appeared to be the inferior therapy should have their treatment changed. This same concern would have equal force in a study with historical controls if they were recent, as has been advised,[5] and the patients are still living. Despite the comments above, ethical problems are real ones and must be faced squarely. There is always some cost in learning something. The great advantage of randomized trials is that we may get a clear answer, and in the long run this appears to be a more ethical course of behavior, provided that the patients involved in the trials are aware of the nature of the study and the reasons for it.

CONCLUDING REMARKS

The only situations in which I would be likely to support a nonrandomized study relying on historical controls would be in the study of diseases so rare that it was just not possible to obtain enough patients in a reasonable period of time for concomitant randomized comparisons, or when a new treatment appears that is markedly effective for a disease which before that time was virtually incurable. In the former instance I would be guided by practical considerations alone, and in the latter situation one could be reasonably certain that the kinds of biases I have discussed would not mask the treatment effect or be confused with it. In addition, it would be difficult or impossible to justify a randomized study in the latter situation from a ethical point of view. Of course those favoring nonrandomized studies usually imagine themselves to be in the latter situation, but careful study would probably reveal that such situations are quite rare. Historical control studies are often useful in providing ideas to be tested in properly designed prospective randomized studies, and this should probably be their greatest use.

Deciding on the design of a study must always involve a serious consideration of practicality. Practicality has many aspects, including cost, time, availability of patients, enthusiasm, the beliefs of the investigators, ethical issues, and some estimation about whether or not the results of the study as finally designed and carried out will be convincing to others. I hope I have convinced you that in most instances a randomized clinical trial is the best approach.

REFERENCES

1. Gehan, E. A. (1978) Comparative clinical trials with historical controls: a statistician's view. *Biomedicine* (Special Issue) **28**:13–19.
2. Byar, D.P.; Simon, R.M.; Friedewald, W.T.; Schlesselman, J.J.; DeMets, D.L.; Ellenberg, J.H.; Gail, M.H.; and Ware, J.H. (1976). Randomized clinical trials: perspectives on some recent ideas. *New Eng J Med,* **295**:74–80.
3. Pickering, G.W. (1949). The place of the experimental method in medicine. *Proc Royal Soc Med,* **42**:229–34.
4. Peto, R.; Pike, M.C.; Armitage, P.; Breslow, N.E.; Cox, D.R.; Howard, S.V.; Mantel, N.; McPherson, K.; Peto, J.; and Smith, P.G. (1977). Design and analysis of randomized clinical trials requiring prolonged observation of each patient. II. Analysis and examples. *Br J Cancer,* **35**:1–39.
5. Gehan, E.A.; and Freireich, E.J. (1974). Non-randomized controls in cancer clinical trials. *New Eng J Med,* **290**:198–203.

11

Quantitative and Qualitative Prediction of Toxicity from Animals to Human

Abraham Goldin, Marcel Rozencweig, and Anthony M. Guarino
Division of Cancer Treatment, National Cancer Institute, Bethesda, Maryland 20014

Philip Schein
Division of Medical Oncology, Vincent T. Lombardi Cancer Research Center, Georgetown
University School of Medicine
Washington, D. C. 20007

THE OBJECTIVES OF A MEANINGFUL cancer chemotherapy drug development program involve the discovery and evaluation of new antitumor drugs in experimental systems and the accurate recommendation of these compounds for clinical trial. Once a new antitumor agent has been demonstrated to be of sufficient interest, based on detailed evaluation in one or more tumor systems, it is entered into toxicological studies in animals with the primary objective of obtaining information relevant to the selection of a safe starting dose regimen and potential drug risks during the initial clinical trial. In order to accomplish this it is necessary to utilize toxicity data obtained in one or more species of animals and to extrapolate both the quantitative and qualitative information obtained to the utilization of the drug in treatment.

The utilization of preclinical animal toxicologic models for prediction of the risks of drug toxicity in the clinic in the field of cancer chemotherapy stems from a number of considerations:[1,2] the therapeutic role of antitumor chemotherapeutic agents is limited, with little exception, by their toxicity to normal tissues; chemotherapeutic agents exert a wide range of qualitative toxicities; and finally, a variety of antitumor agents exert their cytotoxicity via action upon DNA with resultant risk of teratogenesis, mutagenesis and carcinogenesis. These risks are magnified because: (a) anticancer chemotherapy is increasingly used for curative purposes; (b) in order to achieve a maximum therapeutic effect it may be necessary to employ moderately toxic doses of the drug; (c) it is generally necessary to treat the

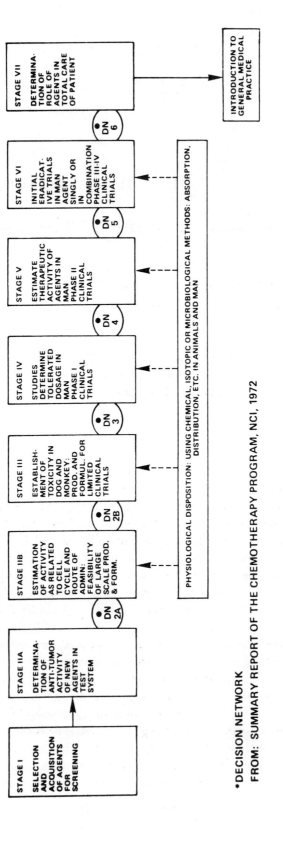

*DECISION NETWORK

FROM: SUMMARY REPORT OF THE CHEMOTHERAPY PROGRAM, NCI, 1972

DR&D, DCT, NCI 3/73

Rothenberg and Terselic (1970)

Fig. 1.

tumorous patient for an extended period, employing repeated courses of therapy; and (d) patients receiving courses of therapy with new compounds may have been debilitated by the disease or by prior therapy, with resultant diminished tolerance to drug toxicity.

Despite the great importance of preclinical toxicologic studies in animals, there has not been extensive systematic study of the subject. The large body of information that has been obtained concerning the toxicity of new antitumor agents in animals, in compliance with the requirements of the federal regulatory agencies, provides an opportunity to analyze these data with respect to overall usefulness for the clinic.

A comprehensive preclinical toxicologic protocol has been developed at the National Cancer Institute[3,4] as part of the Linear Array Program[5] (Fig. 1) for the developmental flow of new drugs to the clinic. Incorporated in stage 3 of the Linear Array is the establishment of toxicity in dog and monkey and the production and formulation of drugs for limited clinical trials.

The range of preclinical toxicologic testing[4] involves a series of steps that are carried out after preliminary studies designed to confirm the identity of the test compound and to insure its conformance to criteria of purity.

SINGLE DOSE STUDY IN MICE

The purpose of this study is to determine the LD_{10}, LD_{50}, and LD_{90}, and the slope of the dose-response curve. The dose-mortality experiments are conducted with male and female mice using parenteral and oral routes of administration. The time and nature of the death is noted and gross and histopathological examinations are performed on moribund mice as well as immediately postmortem. Mouse toxicity studies have been conducted on a routine basis only since 1974.

STUDIES IN DOGS AND MONKEYS

Studies in these large animals are conducted in order to meet the requirements of the United States Food and Drug Administration. All of the drugs in the chemotherapy program are studied both in the rhesus monkey and the beagle hound, employing a standard toxicologic protocol (Table I).

Routinely, both male and female animals are included in each study group. Half of the animals are sacrificed 24 hours after the last treatment, while the other animals are allowed at least 45 days following the last treatment to recover from drug effects or to demonstrate signs of delayed toxicity.

One of the major objectives of these studies is to attempt to define the highest nontoxic dose ($HNTD$), the toxic dose low (TDL), the toxic dose high (TDH), and lethal dose (LD) for single dose and five consecutive daily treatments. $HNTD$ is the highest dose at which no hematologic, chemical, clinical, or pathologic drug-induced alterations occur. Doubling this dose produces the aforementioned alterations. TDL is the lowest dose to produce drug-induced pathologic alterations in hematologic, chemical, clinical, or morphologic

TABLE I
NCI Toxicology Protocol in Dogs and Monkeys

1. Single dose in dogs
2. Five consecutive daily treatments in dogs
3. Five consecutive daily treatments in monkeys
4. Five consecutive daily treatments, nine days rest, repeated for three treatment periods in dogs
5. Schedule dependency studies in dogs:
   (a) Forty-eight hour IV infusion weekly for six weeks
   (b) Treatment every six hours for 48 hours, every week for six weeks
   (c) Single dose once a week for six weeks
   (d) Ten consecutive daily treatments

parameters; doubling this dose produces no lethality. *TDH* is the dose that produces drug-induced pathologic alterations in hematologic, chemical, clinical, or morphologic parameters. Doubling this dose produces lethality. The *LD* is the lowest dose to produce drug-induced death in any animals during the treatment or observation period.

In addition, these studies provide information on the major organ toxicity in both species and identify the most adequate predictive test parameters. The predictability and the reversibility of acute or delayed toxic effects may be determined, and the consistency of quantitative and qualitative observations may be compared within and between species. The influence of dosage schedule on drug toxicity is also studied.

This extensive toxicologic protocol has been accepted by the Food and Drug Administration and has served as a model for the study of the preclinical toxicologic characteristics of new anticancer agents. Important questions may be addressed concerning such protocols. To what extent do these protocols provide information concerning safety in the clinical introduction of a new antitumor agent and to what extent do they help evaluate safely the clinical toxicology of new drugs? Is each phase of the program actually required for the safe introduction of a new compound into clinical testing? What is the cost/benefit ratio of this highly extensive and time-consuming testing in animals? Is it possible to streamline the preclinical toxicologic program with respect to time and monetary expenditure? Should other approaches be investigated? Increasing knowledge and experience in drug development of anticancer agents make necessary continuous reexamination of these questions.

STARTING DOSE FOR PHASE I CLINICAL TRIALS

A detailed tudy was conducted by Freireich et al.[6] to compare quantitatively the toxicity of 18 anticancer agents in the mouse, rat, hamster, dog, monkey, and man. Data were corrected to a uniform schedule of daily treatment for five consecutive days. The general conclusion was that the experimental test systems used to evaluate the toxicity of potential anticancer drugs correlate remarkably closely with the results in man. They determined, in an extension of studies of Pinkel,[7] that, on an mg per square meter of body surface area (mg/M^2) basis, the maximum tolerated dose (*MTD*) was the same in each of the animal

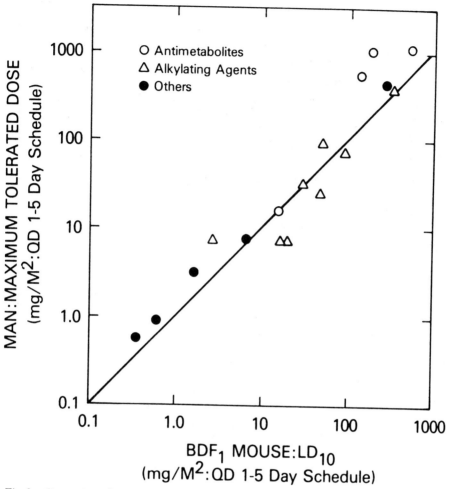

Fig. 2. Comparison of toxicity of anticancer agents for the mouse and man (on a mg/M^2 basis).

species and in man. This finding indicated that all animal species included in that analysis were equally relevant for the prediction of the MTD in man. On an mg/kg basis, the MTD in man was about $\frac{1}{12}$ the LD_{10} in mice, $\frac{1}{9}$ the LD_{10} in hamsters, $\frac{1}{7}$ the LD_{10} in rats, $\frac{1}{3}$ the MTD in rhesus monkeys, and $\frac{1}{2}$ the MTD in dogs.

A comparison was made of toxicity data of anticancer agents for mouse and man on an mg/M^2 basis. After logarithmic transformation of the data, there was a 1:1 linear relationship between LD_{10} in mice and MTD in man (Fig. 2). Similarly, MTD in dogs and MTD in monkeys correlated well with MTD in man on an mg/M^2 basis, and an identical 1:1 linear relationship could be established between these parameters.

Using fixed conversion factors (Km), units can be changed from mg/M^2 to mg/kg, and the correlations on a mg/kg basis between LD_{10} in mice ($Km = 3$) and MTD in man ($Km = 37$) can be easily derived from the preceding data. As expected, the correlation remains

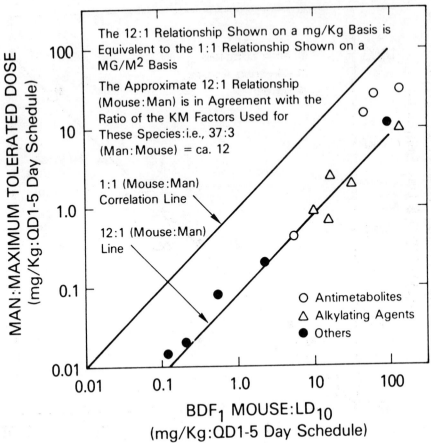

The 12:1 Relationship Shown on a mg/Kg Basis is Equivalent to the 1:1 Relationship Shown on a MG/M^2 Basis

The Approximate 12:1 Relationship (Mouse:Man) is in Agreement with the Ratio of the KM Factors Used for These Species:i.e., 37:3 (Man:Mouse) = ca. 12

1:1 (Mouse:Man) Correlation Line

12:1 (Mouse:Man) Line

○ Antimetabolites
△ Alkylating Agents
● Others

MAN:MAXIMUM TOLERATED DOSE (mg/Kg:QD1-5 Day Schedule)

BDF$_1$ MOUSE:LD$_{10}$ (mg/Kg:QD1-5 Day Schedule)

Fig. 3.   Comparison of toxicity of anticancer agents for the mouse and man (on a mg/kg basis).

linear and is represented by a parallel shifted to the right because of the logarithmic transformation of the data and greater Km in man than in mice (Fig. 3).

Homan[8,9] extended the studies of Freireich et al.,[6] using primarily data of Schein.[10] Homan tabulated the MTD of 37 anticancer drugs for monkey, dog, and man. He used Schein's definition for MTD as "the dose which produced only minimal reversible toxicity," whereas Freireich et al.[6] considered, as MTD, the highest dose killing none of the animals under investigation. With the additional data, a linear relationship was confirmed between MTD in man and MTD in dog or monkey. On a mg/M^2 basis, the regression lines for dog and monkey as compared to man were similar and, surprisingly, prediction from the more sensitive species provided only a slightly greater margin of safety than either one of the species alone (Fig. 4). Of note, the slope of the regression lines also approximated 45 degrees, but there was no strict 1:1 relationship, and these lines were shifted to the left as compared to the origin of the axes. This difference with the data reported by Freireich et al.[6] could be related to a lower MTD defined for dogs and monkeys in Homan's analysis.

When units are expressed in mg/kg there is a shift to the right of the regression lines, and this shift is greater for the monkey than for the dog, because the Km used in the dog (Km

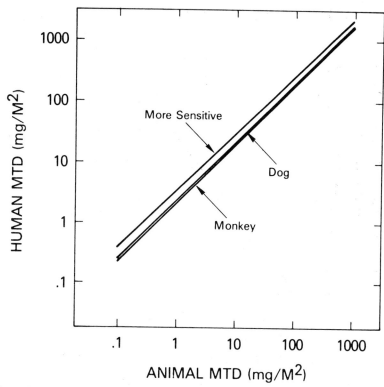

Fig. 4. Relationship between *MTDs* in humans and experimental animals based on mg/m² doses. Lines obtained from least-squares regression analyses.

= 20) is intermediate between man (*Km* = 37) and monkey (*Km* = 12). Comparison of the data on an mg/kg basis led to the conclusion that the dog was more sensitive than the monkey.

In fact, Homan arrived at an estimate of the clinical risk when the dosage in man was based on the animal data in monkey or dog or the more sensitive of these two. The probability of exceeding the human *MTD* was plotted against the ratio of the clinical dose to the animal *MTD* in mg/M^2 (Fig. 5). The clinical risk for a designated ratio of clinical dose to animal *MTD* was slightly greater for monkey than for dog, and where the data were presented on the basis of the more sensitive species, the line was closer to that observed for the dog.

A specific example may be cited (Table II). In general, it has been the practice to use ⅓ of the toxic dose low (*TDL*) expressed in mg/M^2 in the most sensitive species of the dog or monkey. This *TDL* corresponds to the definition of the *MTD* used by Homan. Using the dog or the monkey data carries the same risk of 10% of exceeding the *MTD* in man, whereas using the most sensitive species minimally decreases this risk to 6%.

The determination of a safe dose for Phase I clinical trials was investigated further by Goldsmith et al.[11] They conducted a retrospective analysis of the ability of mouse, dog, and monkey to predict for quantitative toxicity of 30 anticancer agents, including some agents

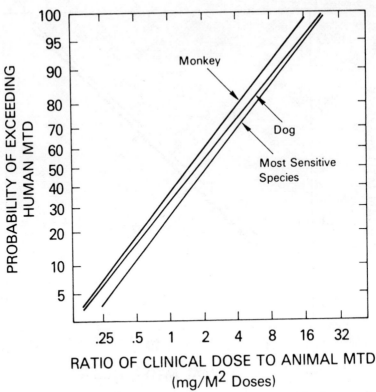

Fig. 5. Regression analyses of estimated clinical risk on drug dosage, calculated as fractions of mg/M^2 MTD from studies in monkey, in dog, or in the more sensitive of the two animal species.

already incorporated in the aforementioned analyses of Freireich et al.[6] or Homan.[8] When this retrospective analysis is applied to drugs where the data are available in all three species, $\frac{1}{3} LD_{10}$ in mouse appears to be a reasonably good and perhaps even better quantitative predictor for human toxicity as compared with $\frac{1}{3} TDL$ in the large animals (Table III).

TABLE II
Probability of Exceeding Clinical MTD[a]

Basis of comparison	Experimental animal	Animal MTD fraction	Probability of exceeding human MTD
mg/kg	Dog	0.1	4.1%
	Monkey	0.1	8.7
	More Sensitive	0.1	2.9
mg/M^2	Dog	0.1	1.3
		0.33	10.0
	Monkey	0.1	1.1
		0.33	9.7
	More Sensitive	0.1	0.5
		0.33	5.9

[a] With doses calculated as fractions of animal MTD.

TABLE III
Ratios of Human Clinical Dose to Various Animal Doses[11]

Drugs[a]	$\dfrac{\text{Human dose}}{\frac{1}{3}\ TDL \text{ in dog}}$	$\dfrac{\text{Human dose}}{\frac{1}{3}\ TDL \text{ in monkey}}$	$\dfrac{\text{Human dose}}{\frac{1}{3}\ LD_{10} \text{ in mice}}$
BCNU	2.7	1.8	6.3
CCNU	9.6	16.2	2.1
MeCCNU	5.4	4.5	4.5
6 MP-riboside	4.2	0.6	3.0
Bleomycin	3.3	14.1	0.6
Methyl-GAG	8.7	6.9	5.1
Comptothecin	6.9	4.2	5.1

[a] Drugs for which TDL in dog, TDL in monkey and LD_{10} in mice were available.

The analysis was extended further by Guarino,[12] in which he included 56 drugs (Table IV). Dangerous toxicity, namely a toxicity ratio (TR) of the human MTD to $\frac{1}{3}$ of the mouse LD_{10} of less than one occurred in 14% of the cases. For large animals (primarily dogs), where the TR was the human MTD to $\frac{1}{3}$ of the TDL in animals, there was prediction of dangerous toxicity in 12% of the cases. With the combination of mice and large animals there was no prediction of dangerous toxicity as a starting dose for any of the drugs.

The question could be raised in the above type of analysis as to the validity of the comparison of ratios involving arbitrary fractional values of dog, mouse, and monkey toxicity. Clearly the incidence of prediction of dangerous toxicity could be reduced towards zero by progressive reduction of the dosage fraction for each animal species to an appropriate level. This, then, would be an priori argument that the dog, monkey, or mouse is acceptable as a predictive model, particularly since the MTD in man is probably very similar to the MTD in dog and monkey or the LD_{10} in mouse.

Thus, by and large it would appear that there is no great advantage from a quantitative point of view in employing one species instead of another for predicting starting doses in man. It is clear that if the most sensitive species determines the starting dose in man, the greater the number of species, the lower the starting dose and the greater the chance of starting below the MTD in man. However, strikingly, the data suggest that the monkey

TABLE IV
Quantitative Predictiveness for Mouse and Large Animal Toxicity Seen in Man[b]

Species (number of drug schedules)	Dangerous toxicity ($TR < 1$)[a]	Reasonable toxicity ($TR = 1$–10)	Inefficient toxicity ($TR = >10$)
Mice (56)	14	70	16
Large animals (50)	12	62	26
Combination (22)	0	73	27

[a] TR is the ratio of the clinical dose to $\frac{1}{3}\ LD_{10}$ in mouse or $\frac{1}{3}\ MTD$ in large animals.
[b] Guarino, A.M. *Methods in Cancer Research*, Academic Press, New York (in Press).

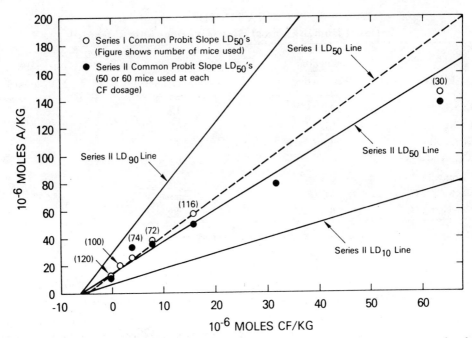

Fig. 6. Linear relationship between LD_{50} of aminopterin and added CF from the fitted modified probit plane for Series I and II: LD_{10} and LD_{90} lines for Series II.

does not add much to the information that may be obtained in the dog alone[8] whereas, along the same line, dog and mouse (and monkey) appear superior to dog (and monkey).[12] Possibly, the best combination would be the utilization of combined toxicity data in the mouse and dog for each new drug of interest.

The mouse could be a prime target for quantitative toxicologic evaluation. It is possible with the mouse to use a large number of animals in the design of experiments involving dose-response relationships, with the establishment of accurate dose-response curves. In

TABLE V
Maximum Likelihood Estimates of Parameters[a]

	Series I	Series II
LD_{50} inhibition index[b] $K_{50} = A_{50}/(C + CF)$ *Ratio of LD_{50} of aminopterin in moles/kg to added plus endogenous equivalent of CF in mol/kg.*	2.72 ± 0.25^c	2.28 ± 0.27^c
Endogenous reserve equivalent $= C$ 10^{-6} mol CF/kg	4.89 ± 0.75	6.03 ± 1.29
Probit slope $= b$ Probits per 10-fold increase in $A/(C + CF)$.	4.13 ± 0.23	4.05 ± 0.55

[a] Relating probit of response linearly to the logarithm of the ratio of administered aminopterin to administered plus endogenous equivalent of citrovorum factor (modified probit plane).
[b] Equivalent to increase in LD_{50} of aminopterin in moles/kg per mole/kg increase in citrovorum *factor*.
[c] Standard error of estimate. For Series II, standard errors have been stepped up by a factor of $\sqrt{2.06}$ to reflect heterogeneity of results.

a short time it is possible to amass a large body of quantitative data, not only in normal mice, but also in mice that are carrying tumors. Thus, for quantitative evaluation, a series of protocols could be developed employing mice, which could be highly useful in the investigation of dose-response relationships with respect to routes and schedules of administration and other response parameters of potential clinical interest.

Once a safe dose has been established in the clinic, detailed pharmacological and biochemical investigation of the mechanism of action of specific types of drugs in the clinic may lead to the means for more refined prediction of safe starting doses for individual patients. It is of interest to cite some animal studies in mice with folic acid antagonists.[13,14,15,16] The toxicity of a metabolic inhibitor is a function of $I/(S + C)$, where I is the inhibitor, S is the substrate added, and C is the endogenous protection in the host, all expressed in moles/kg. This is illustrated by a study in which the median lethal dose of aminopterin to mice was determined to be a function of the dose of citrovorum factor administered plus a low level of endogenous protection in the host. When no citrovorum factor is administered, the toxicity is a function of I/C, and for the 50% mortality response is manifested as the LD_{50} dose (Fig. 6, Table V). Thus, the tolerated dose for an individual animal or patient may be largely dependent upon the status of the subject with respect to endogenous protection, which in turn might be regulated successfully by adjusting the amount of citrovorum factor administered.

In the studies with mice on schedules of administration of drugs it is also possible to determine the extent of cumulative toxicity and the time required for recovery from drug toxicity. For example, in one study it was observed that in the treatment of mice with two doses of aminopterin spaced 24 hours apart, the drug was considerably more toxic than on single-dose administration (Fig. 7).[15] The LD_{50} on single treatment was 4–5 mg/kg, whereas with two daily doses the LD_{50} was reduced to 1 mg/kg. It required a four-day interval between the two treatments for the mice to evidence recovery from the initial treatment.

It is possible to identify optimal levels for a metabolite employed in conjunction with an antimetabolite. This is illustrated in an example involving protection by nicotinomide against the lethal toxicity of 3-acetylpyridine (Fig. 8).[17] In the lower dose range of metabolite, as the dose of nicotinomide was increased, the LD_{50} dose for 3-acetylpyridine increased in linear fashion. However, a dose was then reached at which the nicotinomide began to exert its own toxicity, and the extent of protection diminished. The occurrence of such a negative slope at higher doses of metabolite would indicate that it is making a contribution to toxicity.

The influence of timing of a metabolite, in relation to an antimetabolite, can be investigated in the mice. It was observed, for example, that on single-dose administration of aminopterin there was a decrease in the protection afforded by citrovorum factor as its administration was delayed, so that with a delay of 48 hours the citrovorum factor appeared to be no longer effective.[13,15,16] However, even with a 24-hour delay the administration of a massive dose of citrovorum factor was still capable of exerting protective action against the lethal toxicity of aminopterin. It is of interest to note that with a 24-hour delay the citrovorum factor could not afford protection for leukemia L1210 cells, and that this differential effect on the host and tumor served as the basis of the improved therapy with

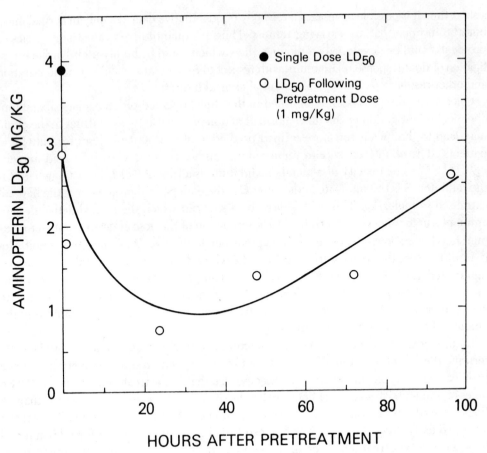

Fig. 7. Effect of pretreatment with aminopterin (1 mg/kg at 0 hour) on the toxicity of a second dose of aminopterin.

high-dose aminopterin and delayed administration of citrovorum factor.[18] The differential protection for the host permitted the utilization of a higher dose of aminopterin with resultant improved antileukemic action. Similar observations have been made with amethopterin plus citrovorum factor.[19]

In mice it is possible to detect and characterize a precursor of an active metabolite. Folic acid administered an hour early afforded protection against aminopterin toxicity in mice. However, on simultaneous administration no protection was observed.[20] Apparently, the one-hour interval was required for the folic acid to be transformed to an active metabolite, and the enzyme dihydrofolate reductase involved in this conversion is inhibited rather rapidly by the folic acid antagonist.

It is possible to determine the relative protection afforded by a series of protective agents against an antagonist. In the protection against the acute lethal toxicity of 6-mercaptopurine, the order of protective ability was as follows: adenylic acid > diphosphopyridine nucleotide > adenosine triphosphate > ribosenucleic acid > guanylic acid > thymidine > adenine.[21]

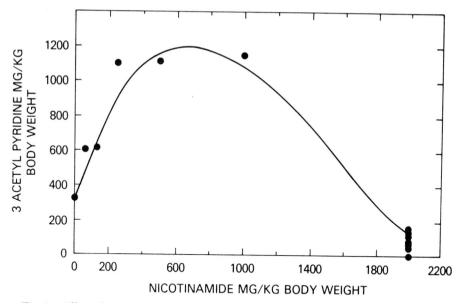

Fig. 8. Effect of nicotinamide on the median lethal dose (LD_{50}) of acetyl pyridine in mice.

Similarly, it is possible in mice to identify metabolic products that may afford protection against an antagonist, such as in thymidine "rescue" against the toxicity of a folic acid antagonist.[22]

Thus, there are a variety of ways in which factors that may influence toxicity for the host may be investigated in mice in a quantitative manner.

It is also possible to investigate the toxicity of drugs, taking into account the host-tumor relationship. In one system, a comparison is made of the relative effectiveness of treatments at equal toxic risk for the host. For example, at equal cost in drug-induced toxic lethality, amethopterin (methotrexate) was more effective than aminopterin in increasing the survival time of leukemic mice (Fig. 9).[23] In other studies it was observed that at equal cost in lethal toxicity, intermittent treatment with aminopterin[24] or with methotrexate[15,23] on days 2 plus 6 following leukemic inoculation was more effective than daily treatment over the same interval in increasing the survival time of the leukemic animals. This was attributable to the ability to reach a higher total dosage of the drug on the intermittent treatment schedule (Fig. 10). Apparently, with the intermittent schedule (days 2 plus 6) the host recovered sufficiently so that it could tolerate a higher dosage of the drug, whereas the tumor cell population did not recover as extensively.

As indicated above, at equal risk in lethal mortality aminopterin plus delayed administration of citrovorum factor was more effective in the treatment of leukemia L1210 than aminopterin alone (Fig. 11).

In still another study, it was possible to demonstrate that at equal risk in lethal mortality, intermittent treatment with aminopterin plus delayed administration of citrovorum factor resulted in further therapeutic advantage.[25] With this treatment modality the increase in

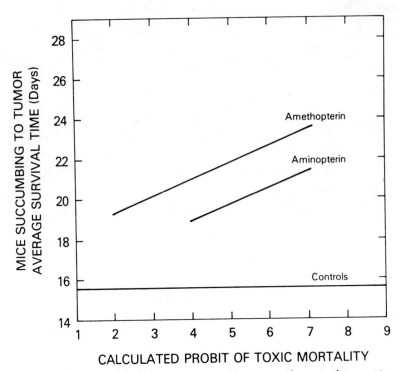

Fig. 9. Effect of administration of aminopterin and of amethopterin on the survival time-toxic mortality relationship in leukemic mice. Inoculum 99,000 cells per mouse. Drug treatment three days following tumor inoculation. Least-squares relationships between time to death from tumor for mice surviving aminopterin or
amethopterin toxicity and the calculated probit of toxic mortality for the drugs were fitted. Separate common-
slope lines are shown for each treatment group. $P < 0.025$ for the differences in the levels of the fitted lines. Control
line is based on the average tumor survival time for 26 mice receiving no antagonist.

survival time was greater than that observed with either the intermittent treatment alone
or delayed administration of citrovorum factor alone.

Thus it is possible, employing tumorous animals, to take into account the toxicity for the
host and to manipulate it in a manner that will permit an improved therapeutic response.
Such findings may be of considerable interest for clinical application of chemotherapeutic
agents.

Following the establishment of a safe starting dose in the clinic, the question arises as
to the schedule that might be employed most effectively in the determination of therapeutic
efficacy. Should a single treatment schedule be employed, or some form of multiple
treatment or intermittent treatment schedule? Clearly, it would not be advisable to test
for therapeutic efficacy with single treatment if the animal data indicated that a drug ex-
erted no therapeutic activity on single treatment, but showed marked activity on multiple
treatment schedules. Studies in mice may be helpful in such decision making, since it is
possible to determine the schedule dependency characteristics of new drugs with respect
to toxicity for the host and antitumor effectiveness. Optimal scheduling in normal and
tumorous mice may serve as a guide for optimization of clinical trial.

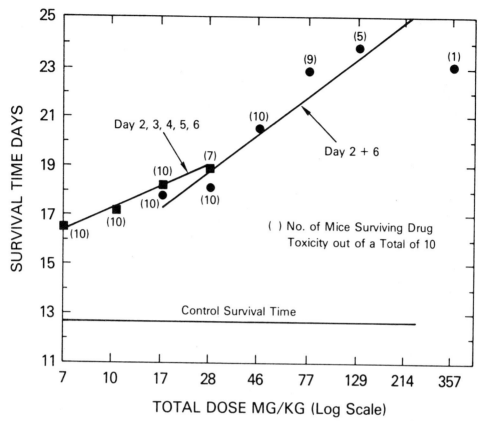

Fig. 10. Comparison of the antileukemic action of daily administration and spaced treatment with amethopterin.

PREDICTION OF QUALITATIVE TOXICITIES FOR MAN

Schein et al. conducted a retrospective analysis of the ability of the dog and monkey to predict for qualitative human organ system toxicity in man.[10] The study was conducted with 25 anticancer drugs of diverse functional classification. The animal toxicologic evaluations were performed under the earlier protocols at NCI,[3] in which only the acute lethal toxicity in dogs and subacute repeated dose toxicology in both dogs and monkeys were determined. In this study approximately 170 parameters were examined.

The dog and the monkey performed equally well in the prediction of leukopenia, with 60% and 61% true positives and 20% and 17% false negatives respectively (Table VI). The dog was more effective in the prediction of anemia, with a higher percentage of true positives and fewer false positive and false negative predictions as compared with that observed with the monkey. The monkey would appear to be a less acceptable model for the determination of the important clinical problem of thrombocytopenia, since with the monkey there were 56% false negative predictions (corrected value) as compared to 19% for the dog.

The dog was the superior species with respect to prediction of gastrointestinal toxicity

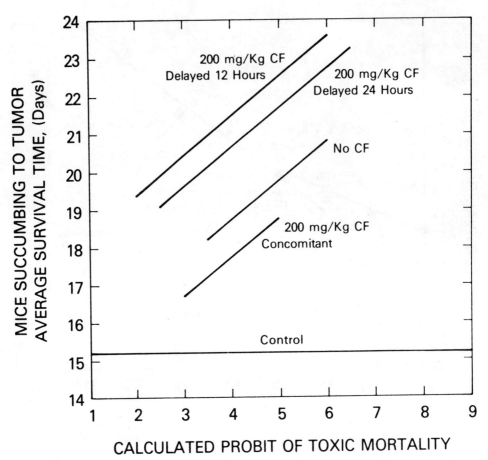

Fig. 11. Effect of concomitant and of delayed administration of citrovorum factor on the survival time-toxic mortality relationship in leukemic mice. Fitted least-squares relationships between time to death from tumor for mice surviving aminopterin toxicity and the calculated probit of toxic mortality from aminopterin are plotted. Separate common-slope lines are shown for aminopterin alone (0 CF) and for 200 mg/kg. CF given concomitantly or 12 or 24 hours after aminopterin. Lines are drawn to extend approximately over the range of calculated probits at which there were any survivors. Control line is based on the average tumor survival time for 53 mice receiving no aminopterin.

(Table VII). It yielded 92% true positives and no false negatives, as compared with 74% true positives and 19% false negatives for the monkey.

Both the dog and the monkey overpredicted for liver toxicity, there being 44% false positive predictions for the dog and 35% for the monkey (Table VIII). There was also overprediction in the estimation of renal toxicity, the dog having 56% false positives and 20% false negatives, while with the monkey there were 48% false positives and 10% false negatives (Table IX).

It is of interest to note that although the large animal screens, in general, did predict for the spectrum of qualitative toxicities for new compounds, this was at the expense of a high percentage of false positive prediction (overprediction). This was true particularly for renal

TABLE VI
Prediction of Hematologic Toxicity

	TP (%)	FP (%)	TN (%)	FN (%)
Anemia				
dogs	44	28	24	4
monkeys	35	43	9	13
dogs and monkeys	48	44	8	0
Leukopenia				
dogs	60	4	16	20
monkeys	61	13	9	17
dogs and monkeys	68	12	8	12
Thrombocytopenia				
dogs	59	14	14	13
monkeys	32	0	27	41
dogs and monkeys	54	12	13	21
Hematologic toxicity				
dogs	80	12	0	8
monkeys	83	13	0	4
dogs and monkeys	88	12	0	0

and hepatic toxicity. This may be attributable to the fact that in order to elicit all of the possible qualitative toxicities for a given compound, it was necessary to employ severely toxic and in fact sometimes lethal dose levels. This occurred especially with the prediction of hematologic, liver and neurologic toxicity (Table X). This practice differs from Phase I clinical trial, where the investigation is discontinued once the initial dose-limiting toxicity occurs. In addition, in this analysis, the most sensitive species was always selected, when considering dog and monkey data. Also, there are apparently distinct differences in the sensitivity to drug toxicity in dog, monkey, and man with respect to specific organ systems. Thus, although there may be a correspondence of susceptibility of a specific organ system

TABLE VII
Prediction of Gastrointestinal Toxicity

	TP (%)	FP (%)	TN (%)	FN (%)
Vomiting				
dogs	72	16	0	12
monkeys	26	13	4	57
dogs and monkeys	72	16	0	12
Diarrhea				
dogs	36	40	20	4
monkeys	13	26	35	26
dogs and monkeys	36	44	16	4
Gastrointestinal Toxicity				
dogs	92	8	0	0
monkeys	74	9	0	17
dogs and monkeys	92	8	0	0

TABLE VIII
Single Liver-Function Parameters in Dogs and Monkeys as Predictors for
Hepatotoxicity in Man

	TP (%)	FP (%)	TN (%)	FN (%)
BSP				
dog	28	50	5	17
monkey	33	45	11	11
dog and monkey	26	47	5	21
Alkaline phosphatase				
dog	33	42	17	8
monkey	15	10	40	35
dog and monkey	32	40	16	12
SGOT				
dog	28	39	22	11
monkey	33	23	33	11
dog and monkey	35	40	20	5
Prediction of Hepatotoxicity				
dog	52	44	4	0
monkey	52	35	13	0
dog and monkey	52	48	0	0

in animals and man, the toxicity may occur with respect to different specific clinical or chemical parameters.

The adverse reaction may occur in man at either a higher or lower dose than in the animal, or it is possible that it may follow a different order of appearance, when the total spectrum

TABLE IX
Single Parameters in Dogs and Monkeys as Predictors for Renal Toxicity in Man

	TP (%)	FP (%)	TN (%)	FN (%)
Blood urea nitrogen elevation				
dog	24	36	28	12
monkey	.18	46	18	18
dog and monkey	24	52	12	12
Serum creatinine elevation				
dog	0	18	82	0
monkey	0	60	40	0
dog and monkey	0	43	57	0
Proteinuria				
dog	9	73	18	0
monkey	0	43	43	14
dog and monkey	9	73	18	0
Prediction of renal toxicity				
dog	32	56	4	8
monkey	35	48	13	4
dog and monkey	36	56	4	4

TABLE X

The Combination of Dog and Monkey as a Predictor for Organ-Specific Toxicity in Man

Organ system	TP (%)	FP (%)	TN (%)	FN (%)
Neurologic	24	60	12	4
Cardiovascular	36	32	28	4
Injection Site	16	36	40	8
Integument	24	36	36	4

of qualitative toxicity elicited by the compound is taken into account. Since increased sensitivity to drugs of animal organ systems such as the liver and kidney has been observed, the question may be asked as to whether it is justifiable to introduce a compound into clinical trial, where for example hepatic dysfunction occurs in dogs. It is certainly clear that the primary basis for proceeding with the testing of a new anticancer agent in the clinic must be the potential of therapeutic effectiveness rather than a detected toxicologic manifestation in a specific organ system of a test animal. Nevertheless, it is important to keep in mind that the testing in the animals may fail to predict important toxicologic responses that are subsequently observed in clinical testing (false negatives). Examples of such cases include cardiac toxicity on treatment with daunomycin, and pancreatitis noted in clinical trials with L-asparaginase. Even though these manifestations had not been observed in the treatment of dogs and monkeys, the question remains as to whether these false negatives may have resulted from inherent biological differences in the animals and man or whether, at least in some cases, the false negative results in the animals occurred because of the utilization of a small number of animals in the toxicity evaluation. Furthermore, the preclinical testing is conducted in healthy animals, whereas in the treatment of the patients there may be preexistent organ defects attributable to progression of the disease and prior therapy. In addition, the patients may receive concurrent analgesics, hypnotics, antiemetics, or other drugs that may interfere with the interpretation of clinical data.

There would thus appear to be no precise advantage in the utilization of the monkey over the dog in the prediction of qualitative toxicities, the same limitations and caveats in interpretation applying to either species. If anything, at least in some instances, such as in the prediction of gastrointestinal toxicity, the dog appeared superior. It is also worthy of speculation that, with the development of microprocedures for hematologic, chemical and enzymatic evaluation, the mouse may become highly useful for the prediction of qualitative toxicity.

PREDICTION OF DELAYED TOXICITY

With the employment of prolonged observation periods following treatment, the animal screens have been capable of predicting the occurrence of delayed toxicity. Examples include the demonstration of delayed toxicity for chloroethyl nitrosoureas and imidazole carboxamide derivatives. It should, however, be pointed out that there is no necessary correlation between the organ systems affected in the animals and in man. For example, with the nitrosoureas, dogs evidenced delayed hepatic toxicity, but in man, delayed toxicity occurred in the bone marrow.[26,27]

PREDICTION OF BONE-MARROW TOXICITY

In general, the preclinical toxicologic investigations have correctly predicted for drugs, such as bleomycin and streptozotocin, that are lacking clinical manifestation of bone-marrow toxicity. The ability to identify such nonmyelosuppressive compounds must be considered important, particularly since most of the current chemotherapeutic drugs do exert myelosuppressive activity. Of note, the antitumor activity in the L1210 system has been found to correlate with the presence of dose-limiting myelosuppression in man.[28]

Exploitable Toxicity

There are instances in which toxicologic features noted in preclinical investigations have resulted in clinical exploitation. An excellent example is provided by streptozotocin, in which the diabetogenic activity of the compound has led to the treatment of malignant insulinoma. In another example, the observation that 1,1-dichloro-2-(o-chlorophenyl)-2-(p-chlorophenyl) ethane was capable of selectively destroying the adrenal cortex of the dog resulted in the use of this compound in the treatment of adrenocortical carcinoma.

There has not been a systematic analysis to determine whether it is possible to predict for schedules of drug administration that might result in improvement of the therapeutic index. That such schedules may be of considerable importance is evidenced by the example of clinical investigation of the antimetabolite 5-fluoro-2′-deoxyuridine, where administration by 24-hour IV infusion resulted in accentuation of both hematological and gastrointestinal toxicity as the result of decreased catabolism and increased phosphorylation to the "S-phase" active deoxynucleotide. In contrast, the dog failed to predict for this marked increase in toxicity of 5-fluoro-2′-deoxyuridine when the antimetabolite was administered by continuous infusion rather than as single injections.[29] It would be of interest of course to determine the usefulness of the mouse for the investigation of the influence of such schedules on the manifestation of qualitative toxicity.

PROSPECTUS

It is important to consider the question of revision of guidelines for preclinical toxicologic testing for the initiation of a Phase I trial for a new anticancer agent, based on a realistic appraisal of animal prediction. The following recommendations would be applicable for the initiation of Phase I clinical trials for new anticancer agents: (a) precise dose-lethal response curves should be obtained in single-dose studies in mice. The data should be sufficient so that it will be possible to calculate relatively precisely an LD_{10}, LD_{50}, and LD_{90}. Concomitant with this, the minimal toxic single dose should be determined in dogs. This information is aimed at providing a safe initial clinical dose and is the most important step of the Phase I clinical trial, since once this is accomplished the dosage can be escalated in subsequent studies to a maximum tolerated dose or maximally effective dose schedule. There would appear to be no need to conduct the initial preclinical studies in monkeys, since the monkey does not appear to afford any specific advantage over the combination of mouse and dog; (b) dogs should be utilized for the determination of qualitative organ system toxicity, both in the initial single-dose study and in a subsequent subacute study. For the latter purpose, daily doses for one to two weeks, for example, with one-half of the animals held for a sufficient observation period to detect possible delayed toxicity, would appear suitable. This study would demonstrate both acute high-dose and cumulative toxicity and would also provide dosage data for multiple treatment schedules in man. Data in monkeys would not appear to be necessary, since such data did not add significantly to the prediction of qualitative toxicities in man. It would be of interest in this connection, as mentioned above, to conduct additional studies of the predictive ability of the mouse and perhaps other rodents with respect to quantitative and qualitative toxicity in man. Ancillary studies in rodents as well as the dog could include abbreviated studies of pharmacologic distribution, establishment of early and late plasma half-times, determination of routes and rates of excretion, and extent of binding and metabolism of the parent drug.

Although, undoubtedly, many antitumor drugs may be demonstrated to interfere with fertility or to be teratogenic or carcinogenic in laboratory animals, it would not appear necessary to obtain such data for the initiation of Phase I trial in the patient with advanced cancer and limited life expectancy. However, characterization of drugs with respect to such toxicities should be conducted prior to New Drug Application (NDA) approval.

There continues to be an important need for research in the evaluation of drug safety, and this should involve investigation of improved methodology with respect to both acute and chronic drug toxicity. Clearly, there should be further extensive investigation of the possibilities, with utilization of the mouse for prediction of both quantitative and qualitative toxicities and determination of the influence of schedules and routes of drug administration, specific organ toxicity, and so forth. Such studies may be useful not only in the introduction of new drugs into the clinic but also may provide information for the appropriate selection of new analogs, particularly where limiting drug toxicity has been identified. It may also provide information pertaining to optimal utilization of the drugs in man.

It is clear that in the final analysis the initiation and the conduct of an initial Phase I trial requires the reasoned utilization of the animal toxicological data plus careful application and monitoring by an experienced clinical pharmacologist.

REFERENCES

1. Schein, P.S. (1977). Preclinical toxicology of anticancer agents. *Cancer Res*, **37**:1934–37.

2. Schein, P.S., and Winokur, S.H. (1975). Immunosuppressive and cytotoxic chemotherapy: Long-term complications. *Ann Intern Med*, **82**:84–95.

3. Cancer Chemotherapy National Service Center (1964). An outline of procedures for preliminary toxicologic and pharmacologic evaluation of experimental cancer chemotherapeutic agents. *Cancer Chemother Rep*, **37**:1–33.

4. Prieur, D.J.; Young, D.M.; Davis, R.D.; Cooney, D.A.; Homan, E.R.; Dixon, R.L.; and Guarino, A.M. (1973). Procedures for preclinical toxicologic evaluation of cancer chemotherapeutic agents. Protocols of the Laboratory of Toxicology. *Cancer Chemother Rep*, **4**, No. 1:1–30.

5. Zubrod, C.G.; Schepartz, S.; Leiter, J.; Endicott, J.M.; Carrese, L.M.; and Baker, C.G. (1966). The chemotherapy program of the National Cancer Institute: history, analysis and plans. *Cancer Chemother Rep*, **59**:349–540.

6. Freireich, E.J.; Gehan, E.A.; Rall, D.P.; Schmidt, L.H.; and Skipper, H.E. (1966). Quantitative comparison of toxicity of anticancer agents in mouse, rat, hamster, dog, monkey and man. *Cancer Chemother Rep*, **50**:219–44.

7. Pinkel, D. (1956). The use of body surface as a criterion of drug dosage in cancer chemotherapy. *Cancer Res*, **18**:853–56.

8. Homan E.R. (1972). Quantitative relationships between toxic doses of antitumor chemotherapeutic agents in animals and man. *Cancer Chemother Rep*, Part 3, 3, No. 1:13–19.

9. Goldin, A.; Carter, S.; Homan, E.R.; and Schein, P.S. (1972). "Quantitative Comparison of Toxicity in Animals and Man". In *The Design of Clinical Trials in Cancer Therapy*, M. Staquet (Ed.) Editions Scientifique Europeennes, Brussels, 58–81.

10. Schein, P.S.; Davis, R.O.; Carter, S.K.; Newman, J.; Schein, D.R.; and Rall, D.P. (1970). The evaluation of anticancer drugs in man. *Clin Pharmacol Therap*, 14:3–40.

11. Goldsmith, M.A.; Slavik, M.; and Carter, S.K. (1975). Quantitative prediction of drug toxicity in humans from toxicology in small and large animals. *Cancer Res*, 35:1354–64.

12. Guarino, A.M. (In press). "Pharmacologic and Toxicologic Studies of Anticancer Drugs, of Sharks, Mice and Men (and Dogs and Monkeys)." In *Methods in Cancer Research* H. Busch and V.T. DeVita (Eds.), Academic Press Inc., New York.

13. Goldin, A.; Greenspan, E.M.; Venditti, J.M.; and Schoenbach, E.B. (1952). Studies on the biological inter-relationships of folic acid, citrovorum factor, and the antimetabolite, aminopterin. *J Natl Cancer Inst*, 12:987–1002.

14. Goldin, A.; Mantel, N.; Venditti, J.M.; and Greenhouse, S.W. (1953). An analysis of dose-response for animals treated with aminopterin and citrovorum factor. *J Natl Cancer Inst*, 13:1463–71.

15. Goldin, A. (1956). "The Employment of Methods of Inhibition Analysis in the Normal and Tumor-Bearing Mammalian Organism." In *Advances in Cancer Research IV*, Academic Press, Inc., New York, 113–48.

16. Goldin, A. (1978). "In Vivo Metabolite-Antimetabolite Relationships in Antitumor Therapy." In *Advances in Enzyme Regulation*, Pergamon Press Ltd., Oxford, England, 65–77.

17. Kaplan, N.O.; Goldin, A.; Humphreys, S.R.; Ciotti, M.M.; and Venditti, J.M. (1954). Significance of enzymatically catalyzed exchange reactions in chemotherapy. *Science*, 120:437–40.

18. Goldin, A.; Mantel, N.; Greenhouse, S.W.; Venditti, J.M.; and Humphreys, S.R. (1954). Effect of delayed administration of citrovorum factor on the antileukemic effectiveness of aminopterin in mice. *Cancer Res*, 14:43–48.

19. Goldin, A.; Venditti, J.M.; Humphreys, S.R.; Dennis, D.; and Mantel, N. (1955). Studies on the management of mouse leukemia (L1210) with antagonists of folic acid. *Cancer Res*, 15:742–47.

20. Greenspan, E.M.; Goldin, A.; and Schoenbach, E.B. (1950). Studies on the mechanism of action of chemotherapeutic agents in cancer. II. Requirements for the prevention of aminopterin toxicity by folic acid in mice. *Cancer*, 3:856–63.

21. Goldin, A.; Venditti, J.M.; Humphreys, S.R.; Dennis, D.; Mantel, N.; and Greenhouse, S.W. (1954). Studies on the toxicity and antileukemic action of 6-mercaptopurine in mice. *Ann NY Acad Sci*, 60:251–66.

22. Tattersall, M.; Jaffe, N.; and Frei, E. (1975). III. "The Pharmacology of Methotrexate "Rescue" Studies." In *Pharmacological Basis of Cancer Chemotherapy*, University of Texas System Cancer Center, M.D., Andersen Hospital and Tumor Institute, The Williams and Wilkins Company, 105–121.

23. Goldin, A.; Venditti, J.M.; Humphreys, S.R.; Dennis, D.; Mantel, N.; and Greenhouse, S.W. (1955). A quantitative comparison of the antileukemic effectiveness of two folic acid antagonists in mice. *J Natl Cancer Inst*, 15:1657–64.

24. Goldin, A.; Mantel, N.; Greenhouse, S.W.; Venditti, J.M.; and Humphreys, S.R. (1954). Factors influencing the specificity of action of an antileukemic agent (aminopterin). Time of treatment and dosage schedule. *Cancer Res*, 1:311–14.

25. Goldin, A.; Venditti, J.M.; Humphreys, S.R.; Dennis, D.; Mantel, N.; and Greenhouse, S.W. (1955). Factors influencing the specificity of action of an antileukemic agent (aminopterin). Multiple treatment schedules plus delayed administration of citrovorum factor. *Cancer Res*, 15:57–61.

26. DeVita, V.T.; Carbone, P.P.; Owens, A.H., Jr.; Gold, G.L.; Krant, M.J.; and Edmonson, J. (1965). Clinical trials with 1,3,-Bis (2-chloroethyl)-1-nitrosourea, NSC-409962. *Cancer Res*, 25:1876–81.

27. Henry, M.C.; Davis, R.; and Schein, P.S. (1973). Hepatotoxicity of 1-(2-chloroethyl)-3-cyclohexyl-1-nitrosourea (CCNU) in dogs. The use of serial percutaneous liver biopsies. *Toxicol Appl Pharmacol*, 25:410–17.

28. Rozencweig, M.; Von Hoff, D.D.; Venditti, J.M.; and Muggia, F.M. (1976). Correlation between experimental activity of anticancer agents and their hematologic toxicity in man. *Blood* 48:984.

29. Henry, M.C.; Blair, M.C.; Shefner, A.M.; and Schein, P.(1972). Beagle dog as predictor for schedule-dependent toxicity of 5-fluoro-2-deoxyuridine. *Toxicol Appl Pharmacol*, 23:532–34.

Thoughts on a Role for Cell Kinetics in Cancer Chemotherapy

Larry Norton

Department of Neoplastic Diseases
Mount Sinai School of Medicine
New York, New York

WHEN EXAMINING THE POTENTIAL for cell kinetics in the design of cancer therapies, we should first recognize that, with or without our direct intention, kinetic principles continually exert an important influence in everyday therapeutic decisions. The ubiquity of this influence reflects the unique place in cancer medicine occupied by cell kinetics, as the final common discipline integrating the diverse intellectual bases for therapeutic growth disruption. Interference with the mitotic process of individual cancer cells is thought to be paramount in modern cancer chemotherapy and is the intended and often realized site-of-action of most anticancer drugs. In addition, many of our most recent activities in cancer treatment research have relied upon alterations in dose scheduling, drug combinations, and combined modality regimens, which incorporate kinetic-oriented concepts of neoplasia.

An illustration of such an influential concept is the familiar and widely accepted view of the drug sensitivity of small tumors relative to larger tumors of equivalent histology. This concept is founded in the often-replicated observation that in small tumors a higher percentage of the assayable cells are involved in some phase of the mitotic process.[1] The sensitivity of individual cells to chemotherapy is linked temporarily to a phase, or set of phases, of the mitotic cycle. If a higher percentage of the smaller tumor is engaged in mitosis, then a higher percentage should be adversely affected by chemotherapy. The result should be a substantial fractional kill leading toward tumor eradication.

This important formulation is remarkable from several points of view. The projection of macroscopic events (tumor regression and eradication) from microscopic observations (percent of mitotic activity) provides a conceptual link between two disciplines—growth curve analysis and cell kinetics—which are traditionally, but not always convincingly, grouped together. Secondly, it elaborates upon the concept of *fractional kill*, introduced and developed by Drs. Howard Skipper and Frank Schabel and their colleagues, and thereby lends flexibility to an already well-established hypothesis. Of greatest practical value, it offers clinical implications that have been widely applied.

The first implication is that a tumor reduced in size with successful chemotherapy should be more sensitive to continued treatment than before such volume reduction; hence, it should be permissible to use less intensive therapy after volume reduction and still cause tumor regression. Also, the application of moderate therapy after volume reduction by surgery should be especially beneficial, for not only should the tumor so reduced in size be particularly sensitive, but the resilience of the previously untreated patient should maximize tolerance to the toxic drugs. Such reasoning, in addition to motivating "low-dose maintenance" chemotherapy for patients in remission, has been profoundly influential in providing a rationale for post-surgical "adjuvant" chemotherapy. In the latter instance, because of both the presumed sensitivity of the small tumor and the concern for toxicity (some patients are, after all, already cured of their disease), the adjuvant treatment is often less intense than would be thought appropriate for the treatment of advanced cancers.

The firm experimental basis for this logical deduction and the impeccable reasoning leading to these conclusions seem irreproachable. In addition, it has been demonstrated unequivocally that volume reduction by surgery of animal neoplasms often allows for the curative application of chemotherapy with regimens not dramatically beneficial against advanced, nonresected tumors of the same histological type.[2] The argument is therefore quite strong, and thence lies the paradox; for the remarkable fact is that our clinical experience does not support the notion that small tumors are easily cured by chemotherapy. Indeed, these tumors often exhibit an exasperating persistence. That many trials of adjuvant chemotherapy have failed to fulfill their earlier promise is well known: in some cases, time-to-recurrence was significantly delayed, while overall recurrence rate seemed less affected. In other cases, even this modest benefit was not achieved. In all cases, the augmentation of cure rate by adjuvant chemotherapy has not met our initial optimism.[3,4]

Although the efficacy of adjuvant chemotherapy remains justifiably controversial, a clearer example of the tenacity of small cancers is seen in the treatment of advanced malignant lymphomas. In many cases, it is possible to achieve complete clinical remission, confirmed by pathologic restaging, with but a few cycles of combination chemotherapy. This is followed by additional cycles at the time of remission, when the microscopic residue is felt to be of increased sensitivity. Despite such treatment, it is not uncommon to see disease recurrences, not because of biochemical insensitivity, but with a tumor still sensitive to the original agents, as evidenced by the reinduction of remission when the original therapy is reinstituted.[5,6]

An awareness of these clinical observations frames a scientific problem of enticing perplexity; to reconcile the clinical facts with at least three experimental observations: fractional kill, the increased proportion of dividing cells in small tumors, and the benefits of adjuvant chemotherapy in experimental animal tumors.

It was in an attempt to formulate an approach of this enigma that Dr. Richard Simon of the National Cancer Institute, USA, and I developed a phenomenological model of tumor

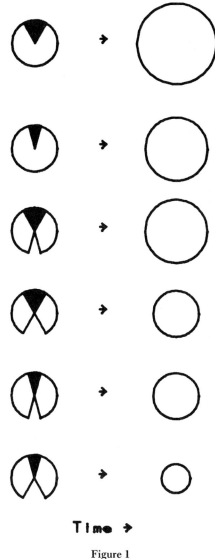

Time →

Figure 1

growth-and-regression, an outline of which may be presented with a graphic notation.[7] Let us represent a growing tumor mass as a circle, a certain fraction of which is doubling in size over an instant of time. If effective therapy is applied, a certain fraction of the tumor dies and is removed from the total volume in each subsequent instant. In Figure 1 the "growing fraction" is represented by the upper pie slice, while the "dying fraction" is represented by the pie slice removed from the lower portion. I wish to emphasize that this growing fraction is not necessarily strictly equivalent to the cytokinetic growth fraction

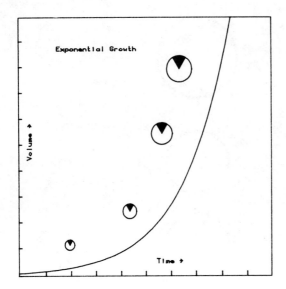

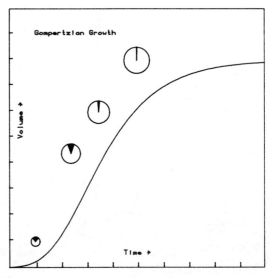

Figure 2

determined from labeling experiments, but may be functionally related to the latter classical measurement in a manner currently under investigation. If the *growing fraction*, or *GF*, is larger than the *dying fraction*, or *DF*, the tumor will increase in size, at a rate equal to the difference in the absolute areas of the two fractions. If, however, the *DF* is greater than the *GF*, the tumor will regress in size.

Many experimental tumors, in particular the experimental leukemias, grow exponentially over the usual size range of observations. In our adapted notation, as shown in Figure 2, exponential growth is defined as a constant *GF:* since the *GF* is a constant fraction of an ever-increasing tumor size, the area of the *GF* (equivalent to the growth rate) strictly in-

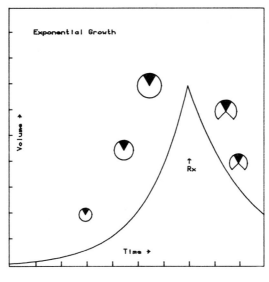

Figure 3

creases in proportion to the tumor size. I have chosen to represent this growth on an arithmetic scale, linear both in tumor volume and time, because this is the scale most intuitively meaningful to the clinician. The concepts, however, are mathematical and independent of these specific graphic methods. When a continuous therapy is initiated, for example at the time of the arrow in Figure 3, it has long been observed that the regression of an exponentially growing tumor remains negatively exponential. This may be symbolized by constant *DF:* since the *GF* is constant, a constant *DF* will generate a constant fractional loss (*GF* minus *DF*), or constant *log-kill.*

But many experimental solid tumors, and most human solid tumors, are felt not to grow in a strictly exponential fashion, but to show a deviation from exponentiality that increases as the tumor grows larger. In particular, although very small tumors may be quite exponential in their growth, very large tumors often slow down considerably, so that a "plateauing" is observed where the growth rate is quite shallow. This is quite common for such tumors as colon carcinoma and advanced breast cancer, in which patients may suffer very large tumor burdens, close to their lethal size, for long periods, with little demonstrable growth. One type of growth curve that fits such phenomena is the familiar Gompertzian curve, illustrated on the right side of Figure 2. In this curve, the *GF* is not constant, but decreases as the tumor size increases: when the tumor size is small, the *GF* is large; but as the tumor approaches its plateau size, the *GF* reduces toward zero. This curve makes intuitive sense if we recall the cytokinetic observation that the fraction of dividing cells decreases with increasing tumor size.

Although Gompertzian kinetics are quite applicable to unperturbed growth, a difficulty arises when we seek a model that accounts for both growth and regression. The greatest difficulty exists in the failure of the log-kill concept, so applicable to exponential growth, to account for common clinical experience. That is, if therapy applied to a Gompertzian

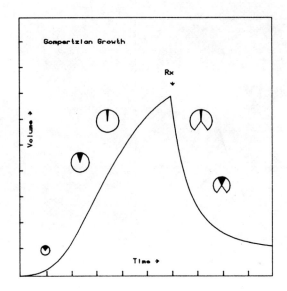

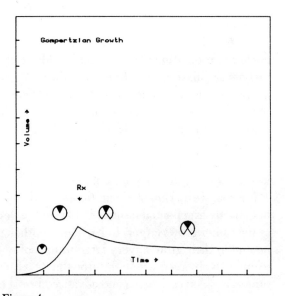

Figure 4

tumor caused a constant DF, then the GF minus DF for the larger tumor would be a bigger negative number than the GF minus DF for a smaller tumor, as shown in Figure 4. As clinicians, therefore, we would find that plateau-phase tumors regress more quickly than tumors of more intermediate size, which is observed neither in the clinic nor in the laboratory. In fact, plateau-phase tumors usually regress quite slowly (if at all) in response to the same treatment that is effective against smaller tumors of the same histological type. Indeed, this forms the basis for the value of early diagnosis in the successful treatment of human cancer.

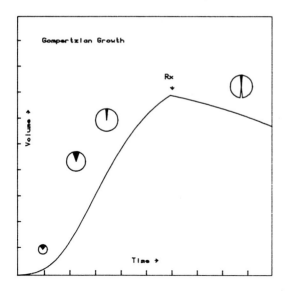

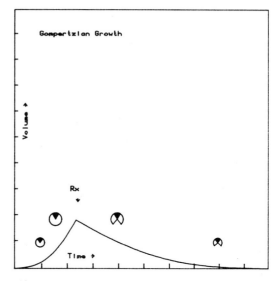

Figure 5

The problem, therefore, is to frame a model that accounts for the clinical facts while recognizing the constant *DF* of experimental leukemia. Clearly, a first approximation to the desired model is evident: in exponential growth, *GF* is constant; hence if the *DF* were proportional to the *GF*, the *DF* would be constant merely as a consequence of the definition of exponential growth. Therefore, if we formulate the hypothesis that *DF* is proportional to *GF*, this would give the same results as the constant-*DF* or log-kill hypothesis in the exponential case.

For Gompertzian growth, however, this alternative model gives results more in keeping with clinical experience (Figure 5). For tumors of intermediate size, when the *GF* is mod-

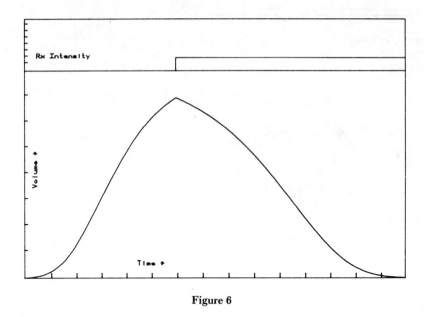

Figure 6

erately large, a therapy sufficient to cause a *DF* greater than the *GF* would result in tumor regression. Were the same therapy applied to a tumor closer to plateau size, the ratio of the *CF* and *GF* remains the same, but the difference in the absolute volumes encompassed by the *GF* minus *DF* would be a smaller negative number: hence, the tumor would regress more slowly. This result—that tumors of intermediate size regress more rapidly in response to effective therapy than tumors closer to their plateau size—makes this model clinically realistic. Similarly, when this model is tested on animal tumors against other models, including constant log-kill, it seems not only to be superior to these others, but quite accurate in both fitting and predicting individual tumor growth curves.[7,8]

It is when we turn to an analysis of the effects of this model for small tumors that we discover an interesting implication. If a constant level of effective therapy is applied for a long period to a large Gompertzian tumor, the resultant pattern of regression is shown in Figure 6. The large tumor with a small *GF* will regress slowly at first, with an accelerating rate of regression as an intermediate size is achieved. This is because in the intermediate-sized tumor the *GF*, and hence the proportional *DF*, encompass a greater total volume. But as the tumor becomes smaller (below a critical point, about 37% of the plateau size), the rate of regression becomes more shallow. This occurs despite an increasing *GF*, for the volume encompassed by the *GF* (which is *GF* times the tumor size) becomes smaller. That is, as the tumor regresses, the *GF* becomes an increasing fraction of the decreasing total size, which results (in the Gompertzian case) in an actual decrease in the total volume (or number of cells) contributing to tumor growth. Since the *DF* is proportional to the *GF*, the total volume represented by the *DF* minus *GF* gets smaller, so that the rate of volume regression decreases. This rate of regression decreases steadily as tumor size decreases and at very small tumor volumes becomes, in absolute terms, very shallow. If "cure" requires reducing the tumor volume below some absolute limit, this might prove most difficult with the time constraints imposed by host tolerance to therapy.

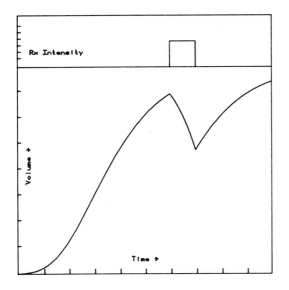

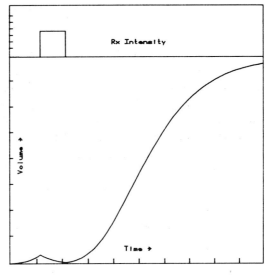

Figure 7

If, for example, a therapy of known efficacy against a tumor of intermediate size (Fig. 7) were applied to a tumor of small size and shallow rate of growth, the model would imply that in some cases the rate of regression of the small tumor would be so shallow that the tumor would not be eradicated. The overall beneficial result may be a modest prolongation of the disease-free interval prior to tumor recurrence. It is interesting that this is precisely our experience in some adjuvant chemotherapy trials. In the case of many experimental animal tumors, however, the growth characteristics are such that a sufficient rate of regression is achievable, so that cure may be achieved with some frequency if sufficient therapy is applied at the time of postsurgical microscopic disease. Contributing to the discrepancy between

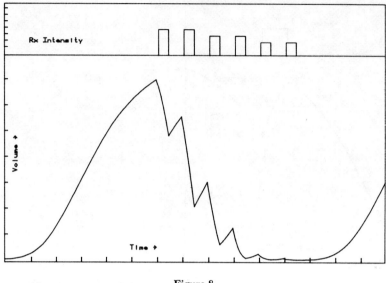

Figure 8

the response of experimental tumors and human neoplasms to adjuvant chemotherapy are the different growth patterns of such tumors as experimental leukemia and the more rapid and uniform growth rates of transplantable solid tumors.

If a tumor is reduced into complete remission by earlier therapy, the application of later cycles may bring the tumor into a slow rate-of-regression phase, as above, which would be insufficient to drive the tumor below the critical level that precludes later regrowth (Fig. 8). Hence, the tumor may recur with retained histology, site, and sensitivity to treatment.

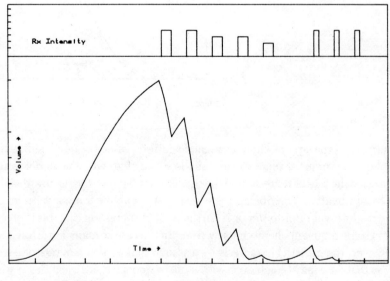

Figure 9

This is because, after all, it is the same tumor, recurring not because of biochemical insensitivity but because of insufficient treatment at the time of remission.

This analysis would suggest, of course, that it may be beneficial to supplement remission-inducing therapy with a brief, intensive treatment after the disappearance of clinical disease, to create a curative rate of regression. A computer simulation of such a plan is shown in Fig. 9. A conventional plan of treatment (Fig. 8: more intense initially, tapering as tumor volume regresses) is not curative, but an alternate therapy (Fig. 9), which saves a spike of intensive treatment for the end of the regimen, is more successful.

The actual implementation of such a treatment plan, of course, would be a clinical challenge, particularly with regard to the toxicity of late intensification after initial chemotherapy. By temporally spacing the spike from the induction treatment, however, and by employing carefully structured dose and schedule modifications, including escalations where appropriate, I believe that it would be possible to design a tolerable protocol. Such marrow-spacing treatments as hormone therapy for hormone-responsive neoplasms may be useful to reduce the likelihood of tumor regrowth prior to the late intensification. What remains unknown is whether sufficient intensity for the purpose of tumor eradication can be successfully achieved in the routine, clinical situation. At present there are in progress several trials in breast cancer and one in malignant lymphoma that incorporate some measure of these concepts.

Which brings us full circle: What is the role of kinetics in clinical chemotherapy? It seems that there can be but one rational role for any school of thought relevant to therapeutics: the generation of testable hypotheses applicable to well-designed, prospective, randomized clinical trials. Indeed, the trials should be so designed that the results are meaningful regardless of the outcome, and may be used to modify the hypotheses, which may then generate a next generation of clinical experiments. Some of our greatest successes—combination chemotherapy, combined modality treatment of pediatric solid tumors, and the complicated treatment of childhood lymphoblastic leukemia—have developed by this process. Kinetics should bear a relationship to clinical medicine defined by this interaction. We should continue to apply our kinetic concepts of neoplasia to the clinical setting, but strictly in regimens designed to participate in an active interchange between laboratory and clinic, theory and practice. In this way we may simultaneously accelerate our evolution toward both improved theoretical understanding and increasingly successful cancer treatment.

REFERENCES

1. Schabel, F. M., Jr. (1969). *Cancer Res*, 29: 2384–89.
2. Fisher, B., and Wolmark, N. (1977). In *Breast Cancer: Advances in Research and Treatment*. (W. L. McGuire, Ed.), Plenum, New York, 126–131.
3. Fisher, B.; Glass, A.; Redmond, C.; et al. (1977). *Cancer (Supplement)*, 39: 2883–2903.
4. Bonadonna, G.; Rossi, A.; and Valagussa, P. (1977). *Cancer (Supplement)*, 39: 2904–15.
5. DeVita, V. T., Jr. (1973). *Nat. Cancer Inst Monogr*, 36: 373–79.
6. Nkrumah, F. K., and Perkins, I. V. (1976). *Int J. Cancer* 17: 455–60.
7. Norton, L., and Simon, R. (1977). *Cancer Treatment Rep*, 61: 1307–17.
8. Norton, L., and Simon, R. (1977). *J. Natl Cancer Inst*, 58: 1735–41.

CHAPTER
13

Cell Kinetics, A Guide for Chemotherapy?

L. M. van Putten

Radiobiological Institute TNO
Rijswijk
The Netherlands

MY TASK IN THIS CHAPTER is that of devil's advocate, providing you with evidence that information on cell kinetics is not necessary for good chemotherapy. Many attempts have been made to answer the question: What benefit has the chemotherapist from cell kinetic information?

A. Insight into tumor growth mechanisms help him to design drug schedules which make optimal use of the possibilities of recruitment and synchronization.
B. Quantitative prediction of tumor growth may help him to design more effective differential types of treatment aimed at cure rather than palliation.
C. Information on the likelihood of effectiveness of treatment may be obtained from data on cell kinetics.

A. These subjects have been discussed earlier.[7] Recruitment occurs earlier in normal tissues than in tumors. Data to support this have been collected by DeWys,[2] especially on cyclophosphamide causing recruitment in the mouse hemopoietic system. This makes it extremely hazardous to repeat drug doses at an early interval; in contrast, the host responds quite favorably to delayed repetition of the drug when repopulating stem cells have gone out of cell cycle and thus are less sensitive to the drug.[2] On an earlier occasion I drew attention to the fact that this rapid recruitment of mouse stem cells occurs after a large number of different types of cytostatic drugs have been administered.[6] The conventional procedure of delaying each further dose of cytostatic drugs until recovery of leukocyte counts are observed finds its cell-kinetic basis in these data. In this respect cell kinetics could only explain what has been shown to be good practice; it has not improved chemotherapy. So far, only in leukemias is there evidence that malignant cell recruitment into cycle may play a role in increasing effectiveness of therapy. However, the data are much more convincing in experimental systems than in patients.[9] Recruitment has been noted, however, in patients

117

treated for multiple myeloma,[1] and it has been noted that a variable degree of recruitment occurring in different patients with neuroblastoma correlated well with therapy response.[3] However, these observations do not necessarily indicate how these cell-kinetic data, giving information on prognosis, may be used to improve chemotherapy.

Synchronization was the subject of a critical study[8] that indicated that the therapeutic gain indicated in a number of experimental studies may not be clinically useful for the following reasons:

1. studies gave contradictory results when applied to different tumor models;
2. gain was not due to cell-kinetic mechanisms but to pharmacokinetic mechanisms;
3. the magnitude of therapeutic gain depended too much on homogeneity of the cell-kinetic parameters in the experimental tumor to permit extrapolation to patients carrying heterogeneic tumor cell populations.

Since then, additional evidence for these conclusions has appeared. Helpap and his colleagues described a favorable treatment schedule with a sequence of 5 fluorouracil followed by irradiation. Detailed analysis showed that the good results initially ascribed to cell synchronization[4] must be ascribed to other than cell-kinetic factors.[5] In this respect it must be emphasized that cell-kinetic manipulations cause only small changes in the size of a sensitive subpopulation and modify cell survival even in the nicest systems only by about a factor of two. This is not much on a logarithmic scale where a decrease by a factor 10^{10} to 10^{12} is needed to obtain a cure. Let us remember that a change in pharmacokinetics, causing an increase of drug dose by a factor of two, is much more important, since it will double the number of decades decrease in surviving cells. Admittedly such an increase is hard to realize, but it may well be that most of the variations in tumor cell survival that can be artificially induced in a large number of different models are not based on cell-kinetic manipulations but on induced variation in effective drug levels.

B. The insight into the mechanisms of tumor shrinkage and the importance of further reduction of survival of cells, long after the visible tumor has disappeared, may be viewed as a direct consequence of cell-kinetic studies. But it is not clear how further analysis in this area can help us, beyond the conclusion that therapy with curative intent necessitates intensive treatment even when no visible tumor is present.

Tumor-cell sensitivity in microtumors may deviate from the exponential model that has been shown to be predictive for L1210 leukemia, but a prediction of the magnitude of this deviation on the basis of growth parameters from large tumors is unlikely to be practically applicable for the following reasons:

1. In patients some variation in growth parameters is often seen to occur between tumors localized in different sites.
2. The need to follow the tumor over a number of doublings in order to obtain a valid prediction makes it unlikely that such a prediction will actually be practicable.
3. Since it has been shown in a number of tumor models that deviation from exponential cell survival at low cell load may occur as a function of aspecific host resistance or immunity, it seems unlikely that these factors may be predicted from growth curves at large tumor volumes where these effects are absent.

C. Cell kinetics has emphasized the sensitivity of rapidly proliferating tumor-cell populations to cytostatic drugs, and this aspect has indeed been found to be reflected in clinical experience. However, the classification of tumors into responsive and nonresponsive types has been done on an empirical basis rather than on the basis of cell-kinetic data.

In summary, therefore, it seems that the study of cell kinetics has elucidated a great number of interesting mechanisms in tumor growth and response to therapy, but has contributed little to the improvement of tumor treatment.

REFERENCES

1. Alberts, D. S., and Golde, D. W. (1974). DNA synthesis in multiple myeloma cells following cell cycle-nonspecific chemotherapy. *Cancer Res.*, **34:**2911–14.

2. DeWys, W. D. (1972). A quantitative model for the study of the growth and treatment of a tumor and its metastases with correlation between proliferative state and sensitivity to cyclophosphamide. *Cancer Res.*, **32:**367–73.

3. Hayes, F. A., Green, A. A., and Mauer, M. (1977). Correlation of cell kinetic and clinical response to chemotherapy in disseminated neuroblastoma. *Cancer Res.*, **37:**3766–70.

4. Helpap, B., and Stiens, R. (1974). Die Bedeutung der Zellkinetik bei der Behandlung maligner Tumoren. *Deutsche Medizinische Wochenschrift*, **37:**1815–20.

5. Helpap, B.; Herberhold, C.; Thelen, M.; Stiens, R.; and Koch, U. (1977–nr. 11). Cell-kinetical analysis of squamous cell carcinomas of the oral region and the effect of a combined therapy of 5 fluorouracil and irradiation. *Strahlentherapie*, **153:**774–80.

6. Van Putten, L. M. (1973). Recrutement, une arme à double tranchant dans la chimiothérapie du cancer. *Bulletin du Cancer*, **60,** no. 2, 131–142.

7. Van Putten, L. M. (1974). Are cell kinetic data relevant for the design of tumor chemotherapy schedules? *Cell Tissue Kinet.* 7:493–504.

8. Van Putten, L. M., Keizer, H. J., and Mulder. J. H. (1976). Synchronization in tumour chemotherapy. *Eur J Cancer*, **12:**79–85.

9. Sauer, H. and Wilmanns, W. (1976). Derzeitiger Stand der Synchronisationstherapie von malignen Tumoren und akuten Leukämien. *Klin. Wschr.* 54:197–202.

Protected Environment and Prophylactic Antibiotics as an Adjunct to Cancer Chemotherapy: How Useful?

J. Klastersky

Service de Médecine et Laboratoire d'Investigation H. Tagnon
Institut Jules Bordet
Université Libre de Bruxelles
Bruxelles, Belgique

FOR A LONG TIME infection has been recognized as a major cause of disease and death in patients with cancer. Infectious morbidity and mortality have been particularly important in patients with acute leukemia who undergo prolonged periods of severe granulopenia. Patients with less than 1,000 granulocytes per cu mm have an increased risk of serious infection, and this is magnified considerably as the granulocyte count decreases further.[1] Most infections in patients with acute nonlymphocytic leukemia (ANLL) are caused by microorganisms, acquired in the hospital, which colonize these patients at risk.[2]

In order to protect the patients during periods of high risk, several programs have been designed to isolate them from the nosocomial flora and/or to suppress the endogenous pathogens. During the last decade a dozen clinical studies have addressed themselves to the investigation of a protected environment (PE) and/or microbial suppression with orally administered prophylactic antibiotics (PA). The technical aspects of the management of these patients, which provide adequate isolation and/or consistent microbial suppression, have been described extensively in the many papers that form the basis for the present analysis and will not be discussed here. For this review we have selected the seven clinical studies available in the literature that are prospective and randomly controlled in ANLL. Any analysis based on a review of various published series has obvious limitations: variation in age and sex of the patients, the type of leukemia, the chemotherapeutic agents used, and other less apparent factors that may influence clinical responsiveness. On the other hand,

TABLE I
Incidence of Infection and rate of Remission in Acute Nonlymphocytic Leukemia[a]

Study	Results[b] Incidence of infection[c]	Remission and survival
Levine (NCI, 1973)	*PEPA* (22) > *PA* (38) = C (28)	No difference
Yates (Roswell Park, 1973)	*PEPA* (28) = *PE* (22) > *PA* (28) = C (39)	No difference
Klastersky (Bordet, 1974)	*PEPA* (16) = *PA* (14) > C (13)	No difference
Schimpff (BCRC, 1975)	*PEPA* (24) = *PA* (19) > C (21)	Increased survival and remission rate for *PEPA* and *PA*
Dietrich (EORTC, 1977)	*PEPA* (42) = *PE* (44) > C (51)[d]	No difference
Gaya (London, 1977)	*PA* (46) > C (49)	No difference
Lohner (Bordet, 1978)	*PEPA* (24) > *PA* (21)	No difference

[a] in adults treated in a protected environment or with prophylactic antibiotics, or both. An analysis of randomly controlled prospective studies from the literature.
[b] only statistically significant differences were taken into consideration.
[c] PE = protected environment; PA = prophylactic antibiotics; C = controls; number in parentheses indicate the number of patients studied.
[d] difference significant for pulmonary infection only.

each individual trial employed only small numbers of patients, making interpretation of results from individuals difficult.

The seven studies considered for the present review are indicated in Table I.[3-9] A first conclusion which appears from these data is the reduced frequency of infection in patients who were treated with *PE* and *PA*. In all seven studies this advantage of *PEPA* could be found. *PA* were found to be as good as *PEPA* in reducing the incidence of infection in patients with *ANLL* in two studies[5,6] and less effective than *PEPA* in three others.[3,4,9] In two studies, *PA* were not found more effective than standard ward care without isolation and microbial suppression;[3,4] on the other hand, three studies found *PA* more effective than standard care.[5,6,8] Thus, at this stage, one cannot make any clear statement about the efficacy of *PA* when compared to *PEPA* or to the controls.

PE alone, i.e., without microbial suppression, has been evaluated in a controlled fashion in two studies only.[4,7] Both found *PE* as good as *PEPA* in preventing infections in neutropenic patients with *ANLL* and more effective than standard care. In the EORTC study, *PE* and *PEPA* were found particularly effective in preventing infections of the pulmonary tract,[7] a finding confirmed in Levine's study as far as *PEPA* is concerned.[3] The observation that *PE* alone might decrease infection in granulopenic patients with *ANLL* supports Schimpff's finding that hospital-acquired microorganisms are a major cause of infection in these patients.[2] In support of this concept are earlier, uncontrolled studies indicating that granulopenic patients with leukemia had only minimal acquisition of *S. aureus* and gram-negative bacilli and infections with pathogens that are spread by the airborne route, such as *Aspergillus* sp.[10] More studies are thus indicated to compare *PE* and *PEPA* further. One might even ask whether strict reverse isolation in a standard hospital room would not

TABLE II
Infectious Morbidity and Mortality in Patients with Acute Nonlymphocytic Leukemia[a]

	PEPA	PE	PA	Controls
Number of patients	155	66	140	207
Number of days at risk	4634	2022	3134	3985
Days at risk/total days	6.64	0.74	0.44	0.50
Mean days at risk per patient	29.8	30.6	22.3	19.2
Number of infections				
per patient	0.66	0.70	0.92	1.06
per 1,000 days at risk	22.2	25.2	41.1	53.7
Infectious deaths				
percent of patients dying	13	—	32	24
number of deaths per 1,000 days at risk	4.29	—	14,9	11,8

[a] Treated in a protected environment (PE), or with prophylactic antibiotics (PA), or both (PEPA). Data computed from a review of seven prospective randomly controlled studies.

be as efficacious as *PE* (life island or laminar air flow room), where air filtration is an additional protective measure.

The analysis presented here is similar to that made by Levine;[11] there is, however, another way to look at the data available in the literature. Indeed, granulopenia is the overwhelmingly important factor predisposing leukemia patients to severe infection; therefore, we have analyzed the frequency of infection reported in the different series in patients with less than 1,000 granulocytes per cu mm. These patients can be considered a fairly homogeneous population as far as the risk of infection is concerned. Similarly, since all the patients had some form of *ANLL* and were treated with modern chemotherapy, they can be considered a relatively homogeneous population as far as the outcome of the leukemia is concerned. By combining all the patients with *ANLL* and less than 1,000 granulocytes per cu mm from the various controlled studies available, the efficacy of *PEPA*, *PE*, *PA*, and standard care can be compared for larger number of patients than those found in individual studies. It is possible with this type of analysis, to express the frequency of infection and the remission rate of leukemia under various conditions of supportive care in a more meaningful fashion.

The infectious morbidity and mortality in controls and in patients treated with *PEPA*, *PE*, or *PA* are indicated in Table II. First, it can be seen that patients treated with *PEPA* and *PE* spent more time with a granulocyte count lower than 1,000 per cu mm than those treated with *PA* or controls. This observation might reflect a more agressive chemotherapy for patients who have been isolated; since chemotherapy of leukemia varied between studies and even within each one of them as time passed, it is possible that isolated patients received more chemotherapy. Nevertheless, severe infections were less frequent among patients in *PEPA* or *PE* than in controls or patients treated with *PA*. This was true whether the frequency of infections per patient or per 1,000 days at risk (days spent with less than 1,000 granulocytes per cu mm) was considered. Moreover, the mortality resulting from infection was lower in patients in *PEPA* (13%) than in those receiving *PA* (32%) or in controls (24%) ($p < 0.01$).

Thus, this type of analysis clearly confirms the impression already gained from the study of individual investigation that *PEPA* reduces the morbidity and the mortality from infections in neutropenic patients with *ANLL*. The rate of infection per patient was reduced approximately from 1.1 to 0.65, in spite of a greater risk in the patients treated in *PEPA*. Our analysis also suggests the effectiveness of *PE;* however, only two studies and a limited number of patients are available. On the other hand, it appears clear from this overall evaluation that *PA* are not superior to standard ward care for the prevention of morbidity and mortality resulting from infection in leukemic patients. This observation is important, since the emergence of antibiotic-resistant strains in patients treated with *PA* has been reported.[5] Such resistant strains can cause severe infection in some patients; in addition, if the patients in whom these strains emerge are not kept isolated, the resistant pathogens can easily spread throughout the hospital. Thus, treatment of neutropenic patients with nonabsorbable *PA* appears to be unwarranted on the basis of presently available evidence, although isolated studies[5,6,8] suggest some efficacy of *PA* in preventing infection, especially in severely granulopenic patients. Recently, a controlled study suggested that prophylactic administration of cotrimoxazole not only prevented the occurrence of infection caused by *Pneumocystis carinii* but also reduced the incidence of bacterial infections in children undergoing maintenance chemotherapy for acute lymphocytic leukemia.[12] Other controlled studies by Gurwith and co-workers indicate that cotrimoxazole might reduce the frequency of infections in neutropenic leukemia patients as well.[13] The efficacy of systemic antibiotics in preventing infection in neutropenic patients with *ANLL* was also studied by Rodriguez and coworkers. It was found that systemic antibiotics were not superior to nonabsorbable *PA; PE,* however, combined with *PA* or systemic antibiotics, was associated with a significant prevention of infection.[14] More studies are probably indicated in order to understand better the possible role of systemic antibiotics in preventing severe infections in neutropenic leukemia patients.

The ultimate goal of the preventive measures against infection in patients with leukemia is an improvement of the rate of complete remission and a prolongation of survival. It can be seen in Table I that only one single study out of seven demonstrated an improved clinical course of the leukemia itself.[6] Schimpff and his coworkers speculated that the differences in remission induction and survival might be linked to the form of antileukemic therapy. It is also possible that in Schimpff's study, the small size of the sample specimen might have resulted in an uneven distribution of some important prognostic factors such as age. As a matter of fact, older patients were more numerous (43%) among the controls than in the isolated group (17%). Isolated patients have had an improved remission rate over nonisolated patients, but not prolonged survival, in a prospectively controlled recent study at the M.D. Anderson Hospital. The authors speculated that unequally effective chemotherapeutic regimens might have been responsible for the difference.[14]

Table III summarizes the rate of complete remission and the survival at 120 days among the patients included in the seven controlled studies selected for this review.[3–9] It appears that the rate of complete remission in *PEPA* is 59%, whereas it is only 44% in controls ($p < 0.01$). In spite of this increased rate of complete remission, the survival rate at 120 days was identical in these two groups, and, although the median survival could not be calculated accurately for all the studies considered here, we have not found any difference between

TABLE III
Effect of Chemotherapy Associated with Protected Environment (*PE*), Prophylactic Antibiotics (*PA*), or Both (*PEPA*)[a]

	PEPA	*PE*	*PA*	Controls
Number of patients	155	66	140	207
Percent of patients achieving complete remission[b]	58.9	53.0	51.3	43.6
Percent of patients surviving 120 days	60.8	63.6	71.0	60.8

[a] In patients with acute nonlymphocytic leukemia. Rate of remission and survival were computed from seven prospective randomly controlled studies.
[b] *PEPA*/Controls: $p < 0.01$; *PE*/Controls; *PA*/Controls = not significant.

the median survival of *PEPA* patients and controls for whom the calculation could be made: these median survivals were respectively 104 and 107 days. Therefore, it appears that the benefit, if any, of *PEPA* itself on the course of *ANLL* is relatively small.

It may be surprising that a technique such as *PEPA*, which markedly reduces the incidence of infectious morbidity and mortality in granulopenic leukemia patients and increases the rate of complete remissions in *ANLL*, has so little impact on the overall course of the leukemia itself. It must be stressed, however, that many infections in granulocytopenic patients can be controlled effectively with antibiotics and granulocyte transfusions. In a recent large cooperative study it was found that antibiotics alone were effective in 68% of neutropenic patients with gram-negative septicemia.[15] There is also evidence that in patients with severely depressed bone-marrow function, transfusions of granulocytes can be life saving.[16] Therefore, prevention of the infectious episodes cannot necessarily be expected to influence the overall course of the disease and the survival of the patients.

On the other hand, since the natural history of *ANLL* has not been greatly influenced by a reduction of infectious mortality that results from the use of *PEPA* or *PE*, infection is not, and perhaps less so than before, a major factor influencing the survival of patients with *ANLL*. We found recently that patients with *ANLL* died as often from hemorrhage (44%) and from infection (44%); lethal extramedullary toxicity from cancer chemotherapy was also a major factor contributing to death.[17] Thus, in spite of satisfactory control of infectious morbidity and mortality, durable remissions cannot be obtained. The limitation appears thus to be the lack of adequate chemotherapy, and major efforts are to be made in that direction.

Aggressive bone-marrow ablative chemotherapy followed by bone-marrow transplantation has been used more recently as a successfull therapy for *ANLL*.[18] Under these circumstances, since cure appears possible, the protection of the patients in *PE*, with or without *PA*, is probably indicated. The same may apply for patients with aplastic anemias, 40% of whom can achieve a long-term survival after allogeneic marrow transplantation.[19] In addition, there is some indication from animal studies that *PA* might be effective in modifying the graft-versus-host disease, which is another major complication of transplantation. This might prove to be another area in which *PEPA* and/or *PE* should be investigated.

Intensive chemotherapy of some solid tumors might also benefit from supportive care carried out in protected environments. Good candidates for this type of approach would be tumors which are expected to respond to high doses of chemotherapeutic agents. Along these lines, it should be pointed out that patients with small-cell bronchogenic carcinoma who are treated with high-dose chemotherapy have higher response rates than patients treated with a more conventional chemotherapy.[20] In this study, the necessity of protected environment was also evaluated; however, the patients treated with high-dose chemotherapy spent only a few days out of the total course with granulopenia. From experience with acute leukemia, a low incidence of infection for this duration of granulocytopenia might be expected. Therefore, one may speculate about the possible further benefits of still more aggressive chemotherapy administered under protection of *PEPA* or *PE* to these patients with small-cell bronchial carcinoma. Further studies are certainly indicated in this area. Current studies of intensive chemotherapy in both adult and pediatric patients with other solid tumors have been reviewed recently by Pizzo and Levine.[21] Basically, they pointed out a decreased incidence of severe infection among protected patients, with more chemotherapy consequently given to them. It also appears that some patients have profited from this approach as far as survival is concerned. Whether intensive drug schedules will significantly prolong the lives of large numbers of patients with various solid tumors remains to be fully investigated. Protective environment should be studied as a part of these regimens. It remains to be seen whether the limiting factors will be the lack of effective chemotherapy and extramedullary drug toxicity rather than ineffectiveness of support for medullary toxicity.

To conclude: it has become clear, after a decade of clinical studies, that protection of neutropenic patients with isolation and microbial suppression significantly decreases the infectious morbidity and mortality. Patients with *ANLL*, treated in protected environments and with oral: nonabsorbable antibiotics (*PEPA*), have an increased rate of remission. However, in leukemia patients, with drug-resistant malignancy, the lack of effective chemotherapy and the extramedullary toxicity of presently available chemotherapeutic agents reduce the long-term benefit from protection against infection.

It seems likely, however, that a protective environment might prove to be an ideal adjunct to techniques of allogeneic bone-marrow transplantation for medullary aplasia and acute leukemia. Protection against infection might also be important for patients who are treated intensively for solid tumors that are likely to respond to presently available chemotherapy. Under these clinical circumstances protective environment should be studied further.

REFERENCES

1. Hersch, E. M.; Bodey, G. P.; Nies, B. A.; and Freireich: E. J. (1965). Causes of death in acute leukemia. A ten-year study of 414 patients from 1954–1963. *J Am Med Assoc*, **193**:105.

2. Schimpff, S. C.; Young, V. M.; Greene, W. H.; Vermeulen: G. D.; Moody: M. R.; and Wiernik, P. H. (1972). Origin of infection in acute nonlymphocytic leukemia. Significance of hospital acquisition of potential pathogens. *Ann Intern Med*, **77**:707.

3. Levine, A. S.; Siegel, S. E.; Schreiber, A. D.; Hauser, J.; Preisler: H.; Goldstein, I. M.; Seidler, F.; Simon, R.; Perry, S.; Bennett, J. E.; and Henderson, E. S. (1973). Protected environments and prophylactic antibiotics. A prospective controlled study of their utility in the therapy of acute leukemia. *New England J Med*, **288**:477.

4. Yates J. W.; Holland, J. F. (1973). A controlled study of isolation and endogenous microbial suppression in acute myelocytic leukemia patients. *Cancer*, **32**:1490.

5. Klastersky, J.; Debusscher, L.; Weerts, D.; and Daneau, D. (1974). Use of oral antibiotics in protected units environment: clinical effectiveness and role in the emergence of antibiotic-resistant strains. *Pathol Biol,* **22**:5.

6. Schimpff, S. C.; Greene, W. H.; Young, V. M.; Fortner, C. L.; Jepsen: L.; Cusack, N.; Block, J. B.; and Wiernick, P. H. (1975). Infection prevention in acute non-lymphocytic leukemia. Laminar air-flow-room reverse isolation with oral, non-absorbable antibiotic prophylaxis. *Ann Intern Med,* **82**:351.

7. Dietrich, M.; Gaus, W.; Vossen, J.; van der WAAIJ, D.; and Wendt, F. (1977). Protective isolation and antimicrobial decontamination in patients with high susceptibility to infection. *Infection,* **5**:1–10.

8. Storring, R. A.; Jameson, B.; Mcelwain, T. J.; Wiltshaw, E.; Spiers, A. D. S.; and Gaya, H. (1977). Oral non-absorved antibiotics prevent infection in acute non-lymphoblastic leukaemia. *Lancet,* **2**:837.

9. Lohner, D.; Debusscher, L.; Prevost, J. M.; and Klastersky, (1978). Comparative randomized study of protected environment plus oral antibiotics versus oral antibiotics in neutropenic patients. *Cancer Chemother Rep.*

10. Jameson, B.; Gamble, D. R.; Lynck, J.; and Kay, H. E. M. (1971). Five-year analysis of protective isolation. *Lancet,* **1**:1034.

11. Levine, A. S.; (1976). Protected environment-prophylactic antibiotic programs; clinical studies. *Clin Haematol,* **5**:409.

12. Hughes, W. T.; Kuhn, S.; Chauhary, S.; Feldman, S.; Verzosa, M.; Aur, J. A. R.; Pratt, C.; and George, S. L. (1977). Successful chemoprophylaxis for Pneumocystis carinii pneumonitis. *New Engl J Med,* **297**: 1419.

13. Gurwith, M. J.; Brunton, J. L.; Lank, B. A.; Harding, G. K. M.; and Ronald, A. R. (1978). A prospective controlled investigation of prophylactic trimethoprim/sulfamethoxazole in hospitalized granulocytopenic patients. *Am J Med.*

14. Rodriguez, V.; Bodey, G. P.; Freireich, E. J.; McCredie, K. B.; Gutterman, J. V.; Keating, M. J.; Smith, T.; and Gehan, E. A. (1978). Randomized trial of protected-environment-prophylactic antibiotics in 145 adults with acute leukemia. *Medicine.*

15. Schimpff, S. C.; Gaya, H.; Klastersky, J.; Tattersall, M. H. N.; and Zinner, S. H. (1978). Three antibiotic regimens in the treatment of infection in febrile granulopenic patients with cancer (EORTC International Antimicrobial Therapy Project Group). *J Infect Dis,* **137**:14.

16. Herzig, R. H.; Herzig, G. P.; Graw, R. G.; Bull, M. I.; and Ray, K. K. (1977). Successful granulocyte transfusion therapy for gram-negative septicemia. A prospectively randomized controlled study. *New Engl J Med,* **296**:701.

17. Klastersky, J.; Weerts, D.; and Gompel, C. (1975). Causes of death in acute non-lymphocytic leukemia. *Eur J Cancer,* **11**:21.

18. Thomas, E. D.; Buckner, C. D.; Banaji, M.; Clift, R. A.; Fefer, A.; Flournoy, N.; Goodell, B. W.; Hickman, R. O.; Lerner, K. G.; Neiman, P. E.; Sale, G. E.; Sanders, J. E.; Singer, J.; Stevens M.; Storb, P.; and Weiden, P. L. (1977). One hundred patients with acute leukemia treated by chemotherapy, total body irradiation and allogeneic marrow transplantation. *Blood,* **49**:511.

19. Storb, R.; Thomas, E. D.; Weiden, P. L.; Buckner, C. D.; Clift, R. A.; Fefer, A.; Fernando, A. L.; Glibett, E. R.; Goodell, B. W.; Johnson, F. L.; Lerner, K. G.; Neiman, P. E.; and Sanders, J. E. (1976). Aplastic anemia treated by allogeneic bone marrow transplantation: a report on 49 new cases from Seattle. *Blood,* **48**: 817.

20. Cohen, M. H.; Creaven, P. J.; Fossieck, B. F.; Broder, L. E.; Selawry, O. S.; Johnston, A. V.; Williams, C. L.; and Minna, J. D. (1977). Intensive chemotherapy of small cell bronchogenic carcinoma. *Cancer Chemother Rep,* **61**, 349.

21. Pizzo, P. A., and Levine, A. S. (1977). The utility of protected-environment regimens for the compromised host: a critical assessment. *Prog Hematol,* **10**:311.

15

Controversies in Screening for Early Diagnosis of Breast Cancer

A. M. Stark

Department of Gynecological Oncology
Queen Elizabeth Hospital
Gateshead, Tyne and Wear
Great Britain

THE RESULTS OF TREATING many cancers have shown considerable improvement in recent years, but the survival rates for breast cancer are no better now than 50 years ago.

Several published series[1,2,3,4] show that, on the average, the smaller the lesion at the time of diagnosis the better the prognosis.

These two facts have stimulated increased interest in the earlier diagnosis of breast cancer. The methods advocated for this are breast self-palpation, routine physical examination by a medical attendant, thermography, mammography, ultrasound, and cytology.

The majority of breast cancers are found by women themselves—or their husbands. As physicians, I consider we have a duty to encourage and instruct women in breast self-palpation. This tuition must be accompanied by an explanation of the age distribution of breast cancer and an assurance that only 25% of breast lumps are cancerous, but that tests other than palpation are required to prove the diagnosis. Care *must* be taken to avoid causing undue worry in women, as has occurred in Britain recently following a series of articles by the media. This is the first point of controversy, as opinion is divided on the value of such teaching.

In 1967, Gershon-Cohen[4] pointed out that the campaign for self-examination, waged for 20 years by the American Cancer Society, had been a failure. Nevertheless, in Great Britain a controlled trial of teaching breast self-palpation to two large populations of women is about to commence.

Quite apart from details of symptoms of breast disease, past or present, a detailed personal and family history is useful in assessing a woman's potential risk of breast cancer.

No matter what other techniques may be used for early detection of breast cancer, a careful clinical examination by orthodox methods should always be employed. Clinical indications for biopsy should not be overruled by the results of any of these other methods.

It is seldom possible to palpate a breast tumor smaller than 10 mm, and in a large breast it may have to be even bigger to be so detected. Unfortunately, even at 10 mm, approximately 50% of such tumors have already spread beyond the breast, and, from the biological point of view, a palpable cancer is a late cancer.

For this reason, methods of detecting preclinical cancer—i.e., before there is a palpable mass—have been developed.

Thermography was developed early in this field. There are two types of thermography, infrared or contact, and they will be discussed in greater detail later.

Over the past 15 years, the techniques and equipment for mammography have improved tremendously. Film or Xerox may be used to produce the image. Undoubtedly, a xerogram gives more information in the young glandular breast with little fat to give contrast, but breast cancer is not a disease of the young. Much more important is the fact that lesions are not easily seen at the extremes of a xerogram plate, i.e., near the chest wall and in the subareolar area. Unless the negative mode of xerography is employed, the radiation skin dose is higher than that of a good vacuum-packed film and rare-earth screen combination. Xerography has several technical disadvantages not encountered with films, such as reduced accuracy at the extremes of the plates, frequent artifacts due to powder defects, latent images, and pressure marks; the conditioning of the plates can be critical; this method is also more expensive.

The prototype equipment for computerized tomographic mammography appeared to have great possibilities, especially as the radiation involved was very low (150—300 milliroentgen). Gisvold's latest report,[5] however, is disappointing. On computerized tomographic mammography fibrous tissue and cancer may have the same density, the spatial resolution is poor, fine calcifications cannot be seen, and without intravenous injection of a contrast medium there was a false negative rate of 31.7%.

Much has been said, especially in the United States, about the radiation hazard of repeated mammography in screening clinics. The alarmist reports are based on extrapolations of radiation exposures under circumstances, both biological and physical, that are not applicable to mammography by modern techniques. The much-quoted groups of women showing an increased incidence of breast cancer[6-12] were all young at the time of radiation exposure. It has been suggested that the immature breast is more radio sensitive,[8,9] and, according to the published work, the critical age is under 30 years. This is not an age group that requires screening for cancer.

The form of radiation involved in these groups differs from that employed for mammography. At Hiroshima and Nagasaki there was total body radiation consisting of neutrons and gamma rays; two other groups quoted had radiation therapy for presumably benign conditions (acne of the chest skin and painful puerperal mastitis). There is no proof that these puerperal women did not have a nonpalpable cancer or a premalignant lesion at the time of the therapy. The women subjected to multiple fluoroscopies during control of pulmonary tuberculosis were exposed to a very high kVp with a much greater penetrating power than the very low kVp used in mammography.

There is no justification for assuming that the low radiation doses used in modern mammography, even accumulated over 30 to 35 years, will induce carcinoma in the woman's normal span of life, especially in view of a latent period of about 15 to 20 years.[13,14]

Nevertheless, we have a duty to keep the radiation involved in mammography to the minimum compatible with good quality mammograms and also to investigate other non-invasive methods of examination, which may give equal results.

One of these other methods is ultrasound, which has the ability to make soft tissue differences visible. In spite of the anatomical accessibility of the breast for examination there have been difficulties in its scanning by ultrasound. These are largely due to the variation in the histological appearance of normal breasts, poor resolution of the ultrasound images, and inability, as yet, to demonstrate the very small lesions which X-ray mammographic screening can detect. This technique has great possibilities for the future, and already exciting results are coming from a few centers, namely Pluygers in Belgium,[15] Baum in New York,[16] and Wagai of Japan.[17]

Cytology can be involved in the examination of nipple discharges or biopsies. A nipple discharge, associated with a cancer, frequently shows only blood cells and debris, and only a positive report is of value.

In my opinion, needle or drill biopsy for cytology is only applicable to palpable lesions. Again a positive result may be useful in planning therapy, but even with a very experienced cytologist a negative report is unreliable because of the limitations of the specimen produced.

We do not use the frozen section technique for a biopsy of a nonpalpable lesion detected by screening, as there is frequently no macroscopic lesion.[18] It is essential to X ray the specimen to ensure that a nonpalpable lesion is included in the biopsy. It has been found worthwhile to take for cytology a scrape smear of the surface of the area of the lesion as located by X-ray of the specimen.

For the early detection of breast cancer to be successful, there must be a coordinated team that is both involved and deeply interested in this work.

We started the screening of well women for the detection of early breast cancer in 1967. The investigations employed have been a detailed history, clinical examination, infrared thermography and mammography—in varying combinations.

The first project in 1967 consisted of clinical examination with mammography when clinical findings were abnormal. The yield was very disappointing—1.4 cancers per 1,000 women examined.

When thermography was added to clinical examination as the initial method of screening, with mammography when indicated, the results improved. A group of 4,261 self-selected well women, aged 21 to 75, were screened in this way; 13.6% had abnormal thermograms and were examined further by mammography. As a result 42 women were recommended for biopsy—a biopsy rate of 0.9%. This confirmed 27 cancers, 22 of which had not been palpable, i.e., a detection rate of 5.8/1,000.

After the first year, women under the age of 35 were not accepted for screening. In a group of 3,543 women, aged at least thirty-five, whose initial screening was by clinical examination and thermography, the yield of cancers was 7.6/1,000.

In my opinion a lower age limit of 50, as in some screening projects, is too high. Of my total screened population up to a year ago, 48.8% were in the age group 35 to 49, and 62.2% of all the cancers found have been in this age group. In the last year the under-40 group jumped from 5.9% to 34% of the total self-selected group as a result of ill-advised publicity in the press, and I have now reluctantly raised the age limit to 40.

I consider the result of an examination to be a false negative if a clinical cancer develops within a year of a negative screening test. In the women whose initial screening was by clinical examination and thermography there was a false negative rate for thermography of 1.7/1,000 women screened—an unacceptable figure. (By this time, I had also thermo-grammed a series of women with clinical breast cancer and found 21% showed negative thermograms.)

Consequently, the use of clinical examination and thermography as an initial method of screening was abandoned. On the other hand, provided women are aware of the limitations of such a regime, with a detection rate of 7.6/1,000, it is certainly better than no screening at all.

For the third project, women considered to be at higher than average risk of breast cancer were selected from the self-selected group for annual review.

Women were included in this group if they had had

1. a previous abnormal thermogram, or
2. a doubtful mammogram
3. a maternal family history of breast cancer, particularly in a mother or a sister and especially if that relative was premenopausal at the time
4. no children, and those whose first child was born after the age of 30, irrespective of subsequent parity
5. a past history of a benign breast lesion, especially if under the age of 50 at the time
6. a late menopause
7. a previous history of other cancers—of the other breast, endometrium, or colon

In this project, 2,684 women, aged 33 to 70, in one or more of these categories were screened by clinical examination, thermography, and mammography. The yield was 24.5 asymptomatic cancers per thousand and the biopsy rate was 4.5%. In this highly selected group, the false-negative rate for screening by all three methods was 1.4/1,000.

Since completion of this pilot study, the yield of cancers in high-risk women examined for the first time has been maintained. For 1977 the pickup rate was 18.5 asymptomatic cancers per 1,000. The false negative rate for 1976 was 0.8/1,000.

During the past ten years, a cohort of high-risk women has been offered annual screening. Of the original 5,000, 92% are still in the project.

This annual review has been most interesting. Table I shows the examination from which cancer was diagnosed. Since the beginning of 1978, women who have attended over the past ten years will not be offered another appointment for three years, if all tests remain negative.

Table II shows the stages of the cancers found at the screening clinic; 75% of all the cancers confirmed were not palpable. All 5 women with metastatic cancer were found at the first visit, as were 12 of the 15 with four or more involved nodes; of the other 3 cases, one was diagnosed the second year, one the third year, and one at the fifth year. (This last woman

TABLE I
Examination at which Cancer is Diagnosed in High-Risk Well Women

Annual examination	Total pickups (%)
1st	40.6
2nd	18.8
3rd	12
4th	6.8
5th	6.8
6th	5.9
7th	4.2
8th	3.3
9th	1.6

had defaulted the previous year.) Sixteen of those with one to three involved nodes were found at the first screening, two at the third-year screening, one at the fifth year, and one at the seventh. With the exception of the last case, there were no involved nodes found after the fifth year. These findings *must* show that screening is worthwhile, with a node involvement of 17.1%. The node involvement of the false negative screenings, i.e., the women who developed a clinical cancer within a year, was 15.4%.

It has been stated that many of these asymptomatic *in situ* lesions found by screening would never progress to invasion.[19,20] With present knowledge, I consider a control group to be unethical, but, unfortunately, we have such a group of 11 women, whose ages range from 41 to 56, in whom nonpalpable cancers were diagnosed by thermography and mammography. The findings were characteristic of an intraduct carcinoma, and biopsy was advised but not done. Eventually, all 11 presented with clinical cancer; 10 had invasive lesions, 5 with negative nodes, 5 with involved nodes, and 1 showed an extensive intraduct lesion. The time interval varied from 7 to 23 months, with an average of 13.8 months.

It has also been stated[19] that the high proportion of node-negative women resulting from a screening clinic is due to length-biased sampling, i.e., the women with slow-growing tumors with a long preclinical phase are those found by screening. The fact that in the New York H.I.P. project[21] there was no significant age difference of the cancer patients in the study

TABLE II
Stages of Carcinoma Diagnosed at Screening Clinic—Total 235

In situ	104	44.4%
Invasive (negative nodes)	91	38.5%
Invasive (with one to three involved nodes)	20	8.7%
Invasive (with four or more involved nodes)	15	6.3%
Distant metastasis	5	2.1%

TABLE III
Age Groups and Pickup Rates, 1969–March 1977

Age groups being screened		Age groups of confirmed cancers
Age (years)	%	(total 216) (%)
35–39	5.9	8.3
40–50	44.9	53.9
51 plus	49.2	37.8

and control groups (54.5 and 54.7 years) has been given as confirmation of this by Zelen. If the cancers in the two groups had been comparable, the women in the study group should have been younger. Tables III and IV show the age distribution of the women whose cancers were found at our clinic—62% and 51% were 50 or younger. This is in a region of England where the age distribution of women with clinical breast cancer, registered with our Cancer Bureau, shows that 74% of them were older than 50. I consider that this indicates that screening finds cancers at an earlier stage in their life cycle.

There are many people who doubt the value of thermography in a breast-screening program. Although I do not have the implicit faith in thermography shown by some,[22,23] with my experience I am convinced that it plays a definite role as *one* of the investigations in a screening program. It is my opinion that many of the adverse reports[24,25] are the result of lack of understanding of basic principles, poor technique and/or equipment, and failure to attend to detail.

Thermography does not diagnose breast cancer or have any part to play in the differential diagnosis of breast conditions in a screening clinic.[26] Guderic[27] has recently shown that by giving intravenous glucose he can differentiate benign from malignant tumors, using thermography. Unfortunately, this technique is not applicable on a large scale in a screening clinic. On the other hand, one of the greatest values of thermography is as an indicator of a woman's risk of breast cancer. For example, over a period of nine years, a group of 744 consecutive abnormal thermograms has been studied. The total incidence of carcinoma in this group, at the time of initial examination or subsequently, is 193/1,000 (Table V): an abnormal thermogram is the greatest single risk factor for women.

The use of thermography in the screening program increases the overall accuracy in

TABLE IV
Age Groups and Pickup Rates, April–December 1977

Age groups being screened for first time (total 436)		Age groups of confirmed cancers (total 11)
Age (years)	%	(%)
35–39	34	—
40–50	50	51
51 plus	16	49

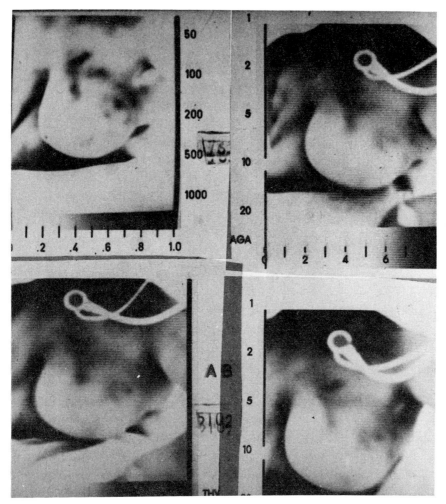

Figure 1

preclinical cancer. Of 51 women submitted to biopsy on the grounds of an abnormal mammogram alone, 43% were found to have cancer and 10% a possibly premalignant lesion. In 125 women with an abnormal thermogram and mammogram, 64.8% had histologically proven cancer and 28% showed lesions of a premalignant nature, mainly very active epitheliosis or papillomatosis.

TABLE V
Percentage of Abnormal Thermograms with Histologically Proven Cancer

Total abnormal thermograms	744	
Carcinoma confirmed	91	(12.2%)
Carcinoma confirmed at later date	53	(7.1%)
Total cancers	144	(19.3%)

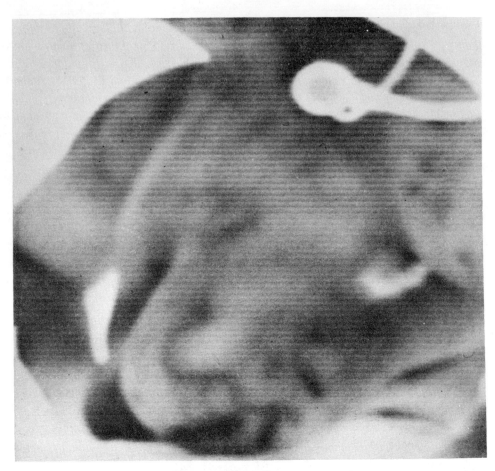

Figure 2

A most useful aspect of breast thermography is that each individual has a characteristic thermal pattern that remains stable, provided her hormonal status is unchanged. When a base-line pattern has been established for a woman, any future increased vascularity is considered a warning, as shown in Figures 1 and 2 of a woman who had a right mastectomy in 1970. The left breast was screened by thermography at each follow-up visit. You will see that the left thermogram remained static over the years and then suddenly became more vascular. At this stage, clinical examination and mammography were negative. Three months later there was radiographic evidence of cancer, confirmed histologically.

Thermography is a passive method of investigation with no radiation hazard, and serial thermograms can be valuable, provided they are done under identical conditions with strict attention to spontaneous cooling in a controlled ambient temperature.

To produce comparable serial thermograms by the contact method is much more difficult, and I prefer and recommend real-time infrared thermography.

Survival rates for the cancers found by screening have not been given. In this context, at least 10-year and probably 15-year results are required. It can be said, however, that to date the survival rates are very encouraging and are *not* influenced by age groups—as suggested in the H.I.P. study[21] in which no benefit appears to have occurred to the under-50 age group.

Moskowitz,[28] however, has recently pointed out that, although there was no improvement in the death rates of the total H.I.P. study group as compared to the control group, the two thirds of the study group who were in fact screened did show an improvement in the death rates in all age groups. Statisticians do not accept this interpretation, however. It should also be remembered that the H.I.P. study was done some years ago and that there have been many technical improvements in mammography since then, resulting in greater accuracy, especially in the more glandular breasts of the under-50-year-old woman.

It would appear that there is potential in early diagnosis to provide a basis for more effective treatment.

I wish to acknowledge the help and cooperation of my technical staff and to thank my secretary, Mrs. P. Hutchison, for her help in preparing this manuscript.

The work is financed by the Women's Cancer Detection Society.

REFERENCES

1. Greening, W.P., and Harmer, M. (1969). Early detection of cancer. *Lancet,* 1:262.
2. Leis, H.P. (1971) Multidisciplinary approach to early diagnosis of breast cancer. *Int Surg* **53,** 3:135–155.
3. Say, C.C., and Donegan, W.L. (1974). Prognostic significance of tumour size. *Cancer,* 34:468–71.
4. Gershon-Cohen, J. (1967). Diagnosing breast cancer earlier. *Lancet,* 1:1389.
5. Gisvold, J.J. et al. (1977). "Computerised Tomographic Mammography. In *Breast Carcinoma,* W.W. Logan (Ed.), Wiley, New York, 219–38.
6. Mackenzie, I. (1965). Breast cancer following multiple fluoroscopies. *Br J Cancer,* 19:1–8.
7. Warren, S. (1973). A radiation induced breast cancer. *Cancer,* 32:991–93. 1973
8. Myrden, J.A., and Hiltz, J.E. (1969). Breast cancer following multiple fluoroscopies. *Can Med Assoc J,* **100:**1032–34.
9. Wanebo, D.K.; Johnson, K.G.; Sato, K.; and Thorslund, T.W. (1968). Breast cancer after exposure to atomic bombings of Hiroshima and Nagasaki. *N Engl J Med,* **279:**667–71.
10. Mettler, F.A.; Hempelman, I.H.; Dalton, A.M.; Pifer, J.W.; Toyooka, T.; and Ames, W.R. (1969). Breast neoplasms in women treated with X rays for acute postpartum mastitis. *J Natl Cancer Inst,* 43:803–11.
11. Baral, E. (1976). Report from radiumhammet at DePCa.
12. Simon, N. (1976). Report from Mount Sinai School of Medicine at DePCa.
13. Samuel E. (1974). Cancer of the breast: forward look in the 1970s. *Proc R Soc Med,* 67:287–89.
14. Crosby, E.H., and Ty J. (1975). Radiation risks from mammography. *Guthrie Bull,* 44:133–39.
15. Pluygers, E. et al. (1977). Possibilities, results and indications of breast echography. *J Belge Radiol,* **60:** 181–96.
16. Baum, G. (1977). The role of ultrasound in breast disease. In *Proceedings of the 1st Annual Symposium of the Gynecological Society for the Study of Breast Disease,* Nyirjesy (ed.), 173–83.
17. Wagai, T. et al. (1977). "Ultrasound Examination of the Breast." In *Breast Carcinoma,* W.W. Logan, (Ed.), Wiley, New York, 325–42.
18. Stark, A.M. et al. The screening of well women for the early detection of breast cancer. (1974). *Cancer,* 33 6:1671–79.
19. Zelen, M. (1976). Theory of Early Detection of Breast Cancer." In *Breast Cancer,* C. Henson (ed.), Raven, New York. 287–300.
20. Mattheiem, W. H. Personal communication, Dept. of Surgery, Institut Jules Bordet, Brussels.

21. Shapiro, S. et al. (1971). Periodic breast cancer screening in reducing mortality from breast cancer. *J Am Med Assoc,* **215:**1777–85.

22. Amalric, R. et al. (1975). Thermography in diagnosis of breast disease. *Bibl Radiol,* **6:**65–75.

23. Gros, Ch. et al. (1973). Semiologie Thermographique des Gynecomastics. *Ann Radiol,* **16:**667–79.

24. Nathan, B. E. et al. (1970). Thermography in breast cancer. *Brit J Surg,* **57,** 7:518–20.

25. Moskowitz, M. et al. (1976). Lack of efficacy of thermography as a screening tool for minimal and stage I breast cancer. *N Engl J Med,* **295:**5.

26. Stark, A.M. The significance of an abnormal breast thermogram. (1976). *Acta Thermographica,* **1,** 1:33–37.

27. Guderic, B. *Personal communication,* Institute of Oncology, 21000 Novi SAD, Yugoslavia.

28. Moskowitz, M. et al. (1977). "Breast Cancer Screening Controversey." In *Breast Cancer,* W.W. Logan (ed.), Wiley, New York, 35–52.

The MRC Trial of Low-Dose Preoperative Radiotherapy in Operable Rectal Cancer

S. J. Arnott

Western General Hospital
Edinburgh
Great Britain

INTRODUCTION

IN RECENT YEARS there has been a growing interest in the part that radiotherapy might play in the management of patients with rectal cancer, not only from the aspect of the palliation obtained in patients with advanced disease, but more importantly, in the possible improvement in the cure rates which might be achieved by the addition of adjunctive X-ray therapy to the definitive surgical treatment of this form of cancer.

In the United Kingdom deaths from malignant disease of the rectum have remained virtually unchanged over the past 40 years, despite great advances during this period in the detection and diagnosis of rectal tumours together with markedly improved surgical and anaesthetic techniques. These statistics have acted as a stimulus to the evaluation of alternative approaches to treatment, since it has been suggested that surgery alone is now unlikely to make any greater contribution to the cure of rectal carcinoma.

That there can be no complacency concerning the cure rates achieved by the surgical management of this tumor is evident from figures published by Slaney[5] from the Birmingham region of England. These showed that in a study of over 12,000 patients, the five-year survival was under 30%. This is probably the most realistic picture of the outlook in rectal cancer in the United Kingdom and this investigation also confirms that there has been no improvement in survival over the past decade.

Various attempts have been made to improve this situation, but probably that with the soundest theoretical basis is the use of adjunctive radiotherapy. When considering preoperative radiotherapy we must assume that neither radical surgery nor radical radiotherapy is curative on its own, although the tumor is operable. Secondly, the dissemination of cells at operation should be a significant problem either in the form of local recurrence or of distant metastases. Those cells which are disseminated, both at the operation site and to distant parts, are likely to be well oxygenated, unless the surgeon cuts deeply into the tumor, and are, therefore, radiosensitive. In a situation which is completely unknown one must assume the worst possibility and accept that the cells may divide daily, which is the justification for proceeding to surgery after such preoperative treatment as soon as possible, certainly within 24 hours.

Low-dose preoperative radiotherapy would appear to be the form of treatment which has the most advantage. Although only a moderate degree of cell sterilization is obtained before any dissemination at operation, there is a negligible disturbance of the surgical field and wound healing is not delayed. Immediate operation is possible after such treatment, and further radiotherapy after surgery is not prevented, should it be necessary. Most commonly, this X-ray therapy is given over a period of days using a fractionated regime. However, studies of survival curves from mammalian cells show that a 90% depopulation of well-oxygenated cells may be achieved with the use of a 500-rad single dose of X rays.

There is much biological evidence to support the use of low-dose preoperative radiotherapy and its ability to reduce the incidence of both local tumor recurrence and distant metastases without, at the same time, interfering with wound healing.

For example, Agostino and Nickson[1] showed that the use of four fractionated doses of preoperative radiation significantly reduced the incidence of local tumor recurrence from 73% to 53% in rats operated on for locally implanted Walker tumor in the caecal appendix. In addition, the number of surviving animals was significantly increased.

Thomlinson[6] also showed that deaths due to distant metastases could be significantly reduced by administering preoperative irradiation, using a rat fibrosarcoma model. This tumor is capable of local excision, and subsequent local recurrence is uncommon. However, distant metastases frequently appear after such operations. When animals received preoperative X-ray doses, the incidence of metastases fell significantly.

Experimental support for the use of a 500-rad single dose came from work carried out by Powers and Tolmach[4] using lymphosarcoma transplanted into mice flanks. A single X-ray dose of 500 rad had no effect on survival at six months, but when the 500 rad was combined with subsequent excision, the result was superior to excision alone. Other work carried out by Powers,[3] showed that when single doses of radiation in excess of 1,000 rad were used, there was increasing delay in wound healing as the dose was increased, suggesting that in the clinical situation, any dose used must represent a compromise between the maximum cell killing which can be achieved and the problem of increasing delay in the healing of wounds.

The principal clinical impetus for adjunctive radiotherapy came in 1959 from the Memorial Hospital in New York, suggesting improved survival in patients with Dukes C lesions of the bowel. Further studies from the same center, however, failed to confirm these initial results. They did show, however, that the outlook was worse for patients with low-lying rectal tumors, those with confirmed lymph-node spread, and high grade of malignancy.

Subsequently, in 1964, the Veterans Administration Surgical Adjuvant Group in the United States began a prospective controlled, randomized trial of the use of low-dose preoperative radiotherapy, in male patients with clinically operable carcinoma of the rectum. This study employed a fractionated dose of radiotherapy given in 10 daily treatments, followed by surgery as soon as possible thereafter. The most important findings of this investigation were those of a significantly lower incidence of positive lymph nodes in the group which had received preoperative radiotherapy. In addition, in this irradiated group, there was a significant reduction in the number of cases in whom the surgeon considered residual disease to have been left behind. These findings were reflected in an improved survival at five years in those patients receiving the preoperative radiotherapy.

The MRC Trial of Radiotherapy in Operable Rectal Carcinoma was started in 1975, and like the Veterans' study, is a multicenter investigation in which 17 centers throughout the United Kingdom are involved. The important difference in this trial is the addition of a third arm, in which a single preoperative X-ray dose of 500 rad is given. In addition, only megavoltage radiation may be used, employing two parallel opposed fields, 18 cm high by 15 cm wide. This field covers the pelvis, the lower border being the level of the anal margin. Surgery is carried out as quickly as possible after the completion of the radiotherapy, preferably within 24 hours. The selection of patients into the three treatment groups has been carried out randomly, organized on a regional basis throughout the country by means of sealed envelopes. Both male and female patients with adenocarcinoma of the rectum, the lower margin of which is within 15 cm of the anal verge, and thought suitable for radical resection on clinical grounds, have been included. All patients should be under the age of 80, be free from any evidence of distant metastases, and thought fit to undergo radical surgery. There should be no contraindication to pelvic irradiation.

Clinical and radiological assessment are carried out prior to the definitive treatment being performed. The aim in this trial, when deciding how extensive preoperative investigations should be, was to try to strike a balance between obtaining the minimum information necessary for a proper evaluation of the treatment, while at the same time, obtaining the maximum cooperation from a large number of surgeons. It was decided therefore, that the preoperative assessment of the primary tumor should be based on standard clinical examination, routine sigmoidoscopy, and barium enema.

Similarly, when assessing possible metastatic spread of disease, apart from clinical examination, the only obligatory investigations are of serum alkaline phosphatase and bilirubin estimations, together with X rays of chest and pelvis. Radioisotope scans may be carried out, but these are not obligatory, as may intravenous pyelography in patients with middle- and upper-third lesions. Surgical assessment has been of particular interest, in view of the results of the Veterans Administration study, and details such as the presence of residual pelvic disease, metastatic abdominal cancer, or the presence of other tumors, have all been recorded. The pathology of the lesion is analyzed from the operation specimen. Its position, its grade, and its Dukes' classification are documented. Bearing in mind the general assertion that the grade of tumors is of particular importance in prognostic terms, it will be of interest to see whether low-dose radiotherapy can influence the outcome in patients with high-grade tumors.

Clinical progress is assessed at repeated follow-up visits. These are carried out every three months in the first year and every six months thereafter. The incidence of postoperative complications, late discharging, or unhealed wounds and residual sinuses are all recorded.

There is at present no evidence from this trial of any increased difficulties at the time of operation which might be due to the use of preoperative irradiation. Nor is there any increase in the incidence of postoperative complications in patients in the radiotherapy groups.

Subsequently, information regarding the development of local recurrence or metastatic disease and its distribution will be collected, together with details of any subsequent treatment which may be given.

Although autopsy following death is not mandatory, it is desirable in as many instances as possible. All evidence of residual, recurrent, or metastatic tumor and its distribution is noted at this time.

Over 600 cases have been included in the trial up to the present time. The input of patients into the trial, from each region of the country, has obviously varied according to the size of the referring center. The largest input has come from the Birmingham region of England and also West Central Yorkshire. In each participating center regional coordinators have a store of sealed envelopes, each one containing a treatment option. When the patient is entered into the trial as an operable case, an envelope is opened, the treatment allocation made, and registration documents and operative details completed, together with pathological details of the resected specimen. One of the most encouraging features of the MRC trial has been the steady rate of recruitment, and there has at no time been any evidence of a falling off of the number of patients being entered into the trial.

As yet, only preliminary data from this trial are available. The operability rate remains in excess of 91%, which is an extremely high figure by any surgical standards. Abdominoperineal resection has been performed in 68% of patients, only 21% being suitable for anterior restorative surgery. The remainder of patients have had palliative procedures, or were unsuitable for any form of resection. Fewer patients have received the multiple dose radiotherapy treatment because of administrative problems in carrying out this option in some centers. The problem has now been solved, but it has resulted in a small disparity in the numbers of cases in each treatment group. The statisticians supervising the trial do not consider that this will affect the validity of the trial in any way.

As yet, there is no difference in the survival rates in any of the treatment groups, but it is perhaps too early to expect any. What does appear to be evident, however, is that there is a small reduction in the percentage of Dukes C cases, from 39% in the control group of patients, to 31% in those receiving the multiple dose radiotherapy treatment option. This feature was observed in the Veterans Administration study as one of the earliest differences that could be detected between those patients in the control group and those receiving radiotherapy. In that study it was later translated into improved survival rates in the radiotherapy patients. So far, no such difference has been seen in patients receiving the 500-rad single X-ray treatment. However, since the MRC trial was started a report has appeared from the Princess Margaret Hospital in Toronto which indicates that we may yet see benefit in these patients. The initial reports from this center, on small numbers of patients, showed that those with Dukes C lesions did benefit from a 500-rad single preoperative treatment, particularly if the tumor was below the level of the peritoneal reflection. However, those results were not statistically significant. A further recent report from the same center, describing the results of treatment in larger numbers of patients, now indicates that the differences in survival are at statistically significant levels, those patients receiving the 500-rad single dose of preoperative radiotherapy having a much better survival rate.

It is expected that the required numbers of patients will be entered into the MRC trial at the end of August of 1978, and already a further analysis of the results is being carried out. It is anticipated that a preliminary report from this trial will be available at the end of 1978.

REFERENCES

1. Agostino, D., and Nickson, J. J. (1960). Preoperative X-ray therapy in a simulated colon carcinoma in the rat. *Radiology*, **74**:816–19.
2. Nias, A. H. W. (1967). Radiobiological aspects of preoperative irradiation. *Brit J Radiol*, **40**:166–69.
3. Powers, W. E. (1965). Radiation biologic considerations and practical investigations in preoperative radiation therapy. *J Can Assoc Radiol*, **16**:217–25.
4. Powers, W. E., and Tolmach, L. J. (1964). Preoperative radiation therapy: biological basis and experimental investigation. *Nature*, **201**:272–73.
5. Slaney, G. (1971). "Results of Treatment of Carcinoma of the Colon and Rectum." In *Modern Trends in Surgery*, W. T. Irvine (Ed.), Butterworths, London, 63–89.
6. Thomlinson, R. H. (1960). An experimental method for comparing treatments of intact malignant tumors in animals and its application to the use of oxygen in radiotherapy. *Brit J Cancer*, **14**:555–76.

CHAPTER 17

Preoperative Radiotherapy for Colorectal Cancer—Veterans Administration Group Studies

George A. Higgins

Chairman, Veterans Administration
Surgical Adjuvant Group
Washington, D.C.

THE VETERANS ADMINISTRATION Surgical Adjuvant Group,* consisting of 26 hospitals, conducted a randomized prospective controlled clinical trial of the possible benefit of giving a moderate dosage of preoperative radiotherapy prior to surgical resection of carcinoma of the rectum and rectosigmoid within reach of sigmoidoscopic biopsy. Over a four-year period, 700 male patients were entered into the trial and all patients have now been followed sufficiently so that five-year observed survival data are available.

METHODOLOGY

In the protocol, patients who were believed preoperatively to have resectable lesions and on whom a positive histologic diagnosis was obtained by sigmoidoscopic biopsy were allocated at random to treatment or control groups on the basis of sealed envelopes by hospital. Those patients randomized to the control group were operated on as soon as possible, whereas those in the treatment group were given irradiation therapy followed by early operation. Following resection, patients were divided into palliative or "curative" categories, depending upon microscopic evidence of tumor at a resection margin or metastases left behind.

Irradiation therapy consisted of a tissue dose of 2,000 R delivered to the midplane of the

---

* A list of the principal investigators is given in the Appendix.

TABLE I.
Preoperative Irradiation[a]

Operative status	Total	Treated		Control	
		Number	Percent	Number	Percent
Total patients	700	347	100%	353	100%
No operation	20	17	4.9%	3	0.8%
Nonresectable	67	28	8.1%	39	11%
Resection	613	302	87%	311	88%
Anterior	183	89	26%	94	27%
Abdominoperineal	414	206	59%	208	59%
Other	16	7	2%	9	2.5%

[a] Operative status of 700 patients with carcinoma of the rectum or rectosigmoid randomized to receive radiation therapy followed by surgery or surgery alone.

pelvis through opposing anterior-posterior portals, given in 10 increments of 200 R each over a two-week interval. Either conventional beam therapy or high-energy therapy was used, depending upon which was available in the individual hospital. When the tumor was within 8 cm of the anal verge, an additional 500 R were given in 50 R increments through a perineal portal during the same period. Following treatment, operation was carried out as soon as feasible.

Of the 700 patients entered into the study, 347 were randomly assigned to receive preoperative irradiation therapy, and 353 were to undergo immediate operation. Operative status of the patients entered into the trial is shown in Table I. The resectability rate was essentially the same in the treated and control groups. There were 414 abdominoperineal resections, 183 anterior sigmoid resections, and 16 "other," including subtotal colectomies, pull-throughs, and Hartmann procedures, the incidence being the same in treated and controls.

RESULTS

At the beginning of the study there was considerable apprehension by the group that the incidence of postoperative complications might be increased by virtue of the preoperative radiation therapy, and indeed in the early phases of the trial this appeared to be the case. However, as the study progressed, it became apparent that this was not the case, and neither the operating surgeon nor the pathologist could tell which patients had had preoperative therapy. All patients entered into this trial have now been at risk for more than five years; observed five-year survival for various groups of patients is shown in Figure 1. Although survival in patients receiving preoperative radiotherapy is slightly better if one looks at the entire group of 700 entered into the trial, a review of the data indicates that any therapeutic benefit is confined to the patients having abdominoperineal resection. These patients received the additional 500 rad perineal dosage and also are those having lesions fixed in the low pelvis and more amenable to sharp localization by the radiotherapist. This

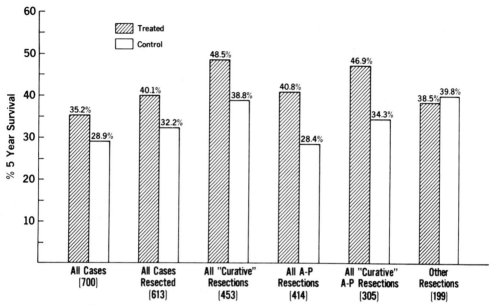

Fig. 1. Five-year observed survival rates in the entire 700 patients entered into the trial (far left) and in various subgroups, showing that the entire survival benefit occurred in those patients with low-lying lesions requiring abdominoperineal resection.

difference in observed survival does not have statistical significance to a high degree of confidence; however, there is a strong suggestion of a therapeutic benefit.

Calculated interval survival (the percentage of patients alive at the start of each successive follow-up interval who survived the interval) provides additional intriguing information (Table II). These data for the 305 patients who underwent "curative" abdominoperineal resection (the group showing suggestive benefit from radiotherapy) would indicate that during the first three postoperative years there is no appreciable difference between the treated and control groups; however, among patients who are still living three years post-operative, 93% of the treated patients survived an additional year compared with 75% of

TABLE II[a]

Postop interval (yrs)	Treated		Control	
0–1	82%		78%	
1–2	87%	57%	85%	55%
2–3	79%		83%	
3–4	93%		75%	
4–5	88%	83%	83%	62%
0–5	47%		34%	

[a] Interval survival of the 305 patients undergoing "curative" abdominoperineal resection showing that the therapeutic benefit from radiotherapy is confined to the fourth and fifth postoperative years.

the controls, while 88% and 83% respectively survived the fifth postoperative year. Thus the apparent benefit in survival in the treated group appears to occur predominantly between the third and fifth postoperative years (83% vs. 62%). Theoretically, preoperative radiation reduces the hazard of spreading tumor cells during the increased manipulation at the time of operation by destroying the cells or by lowering their viability. Thus the benefit would not become apparent until enough time had elapsed for implants to develop to lethal size in those patients not receiving radiotherapy.

CAUSE OF DEATH

Case records of all patients who died either in the early or remote postoperative periods were carefully reviewed in an effort to determine the cause of death and in particular whether or not there was evidence of recurrent or metastatic cancer present. A total of 461 patients who had microscopically "curative" resection (the group in whom any beneficial effects from radiotherapy would be observed) died during the five-year postoperative period, and complete autopsy information was available on 180 (Table III). For the total

TABLE III[a]

	Number	Preoperative radiotherapy	Surgery alone
Total	180	49%	68%
A.P. Resection	122	50%	70%
Other Resection	58	49%	61%

[a] Incidence of cancer found at autopsy on 180 patients dying during the follow-up period, showing that cancer was found in a significantly fewer number of patients having the combined radiotherapy-surgery treatment.

group, all available information was reviewed in an effort to determine whether or not death was attributable to cancer and, as can be seen, this was true in a slightly larger percentage of patients treated by surgery alone than those having the combined therapy. However, in the considerably smaller group in whom autopsy information was available, there is a consistently smaller percentage of cancer at autopsy in those receiving preoperative radiotherapy than in the control group. These data strongly suggest that irradiation therapy prior to operation exerts a long-term beneficial effect on postoperative recurrence.

LYMPH NODE INVOLVEMENT

Analysis of data pertaining to the presence of metastic cancer in the lymph nodes submitted in the resected specimen provided unexpected and provocative information. The incidence of metastatic disease in regional lymph nodes was substantially smaller in those patients receiving preoperative radiotherapy, the most pronounced difference being in

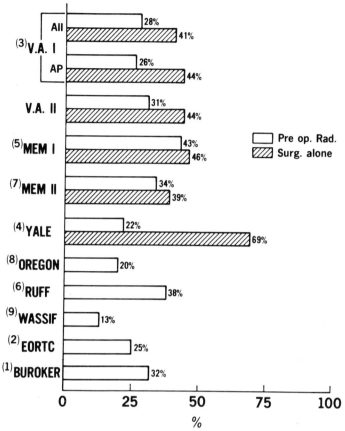

Fig. 2. Percentage of patients showing positive lymph nodes in the resected specimen in various randomized trials from the literature as well as studies employing preoperative radiotherapy without randomized controls. In all randomized trials the percentage of lymph nodes is less in those patients receiving combined therapy, while in the nonrandomized trials the percentage is well below that which one would anticipate from the literature and from the patients having studies.

those patients having abdominoperineal resection (26% in those receiving radiotherapy compared with 44% in those treated by surgery alone) (Figure 2, VA 1). It seemed unlikely that this amount of radiotherapy in this time interval would destroy tumor cells in lymph nodes. For this reason a literature review of other reported studies employing the combination therapy was carried out.[1-9] As shown in Figure 2, this observation has been consistent throughout controlled studies reported in the literature, and in the uncontrolled studies the percentage of involved lymph nodes is substantially lower than one would normally expect in patients having surgery alone.

CURRENT STUDIES

Currently the Veterans Administration Surgical Group is conducting a trial using 3,150 rad over a 24-day period with surgery to be done at the completion of radiotherapy. In this study, only those patients with low-lying lesions which will require abdominoperineal resection are entered into the study. Close observations would indicate that this regimen of treatment can be done without impairing healing and with no increase in postoperative complications. No survival data are yet available, although, as indicated (VA II, Figure 3), the percentage of patients having involved lymph nodes is smaller in those receiving preoperative radiotherapy.

LONGEVITY INCREASE FROM TREATMENT (LIFT)

Difficulties in assessing therapeutic benefit in adjuvant trials in which a high five-year survival rate results from the primary treatment have long been of concern to those involved in this type of clinical research. As an example, if there is a 50% observed survival of patients treated by surgery alone, then it is quite obvious that only one-half of those patients randomized to receive an additional therapy have any possibility of survival benefit. In addition, for patients in the age group for many malignancies, a substantial number can be expected to die during the five-year observation period of causes unrelated to cancer. As shown in Table III, only 70% of those patients in the control group who died during the observation period revealed the presence of cancer at autopsy. This coincides with a life-table mortality expectancy of 25% of United States males of a mean age group entered into the trial. Thus, more than half of the patients who receive any adjuvant therapy cannot benefit from it, but there is no way to determine *a priori* just which patients fall into this category. It would seem highly desirable, therefore, to develop a method by which any improvement in survival could be determined as a proportion of those patients having residual disease who might possibly benefit.

In an effort to solve this problem we have devised an index to determine Longevity Increase From Therapy (LIFT), which provides a more realistic measure of observed survival advantage but does not improve our ability to determine if this advantage is due to chance:

R_0 = no. of patients randomized to receive preop radiation
S_0 = no. of patients randomized to surgery only
R_1 = no. of patients surviving in the adjuvant treated group
R'_1 = no. of patients in R_0 who would survive without adjuvant radiation therapy (34% of 162— Table II)
X = no. of R_0 expected to die during interval based on population mortality rates (25% × 162)

Applying this formula to the subgroup of patients in the VA trial who underwent abdominoperineal resection for cure, these values are as follows:

$R_0 = 162$
$S_0 = 143$
$R_1 = 76$

$$\frac{R_2 - S_2}{(R_1 - S_2) - X} = \text{LIFT} = \frac{76 - 55}{(162 - 55) - 41} = \frac{21}{66} = 32$$

$R'_1 = 55$ (34% of 162)
$X = 41$ (25% of 162)

An alternative way of stating the index is as follows:

At five postoperative years, 66% of the surgery-only (control) patients had died compared with 53% of those who received preoperative X-ray therapy (treated), an observed reduction of 13 deaths per 100 treated patients. Mortality in a similar group of individuals exposed to sex and age-specific population mortality rates would be 25%, leaving 41% of control patients (66% observed deaths minus 25% mortality not attributable to malignant disease) who might benefit from preoperative X-ray therapy by having their survival time increased to five years. Thus, given 41 patients who might survive five years from operation if given preoperative X-ray therapy, 13 patients did so. Restated, of 100 patients who could benefit, an observed 32 patients did benefit; $^{13}/_{41} = {^{32}}/_{100}$.
In algebraic terms, let

SC represent percentage survival in patients given standard (control) therapy
SA represent percentage survival in patients given adjuvant therapy
SX represent percentage survival in patients if only exposed to population death rates
Then

$$\text{LIFT} = \frac{SA - SC}{SX - SC}$$

In the preceding example:

$$SC = 34\%$$

$$SA - 47\%$$

$$SX = 75\%$$

$$\text{LIFT} = \frac{47\% - 34\%}{75\% - 34\%} = \frac{13\%}{41\%} = 0.32 \text{ (or 32)}$$

SUMMARY

In a prospective randomized trial, 700 patients with a confirmed histologic diagnosis of adenocarcinoma of the rectum or rectosigmoid were randomized to receive radiotherapy prior to operation (2,000 to 2,500 rad in two weeks) or surgery alone. Five-year observed survivals in the 453 patients on whom "curative" resection was possible was 48.5% in the X-ray treated group compared with 38.8% in controls, while in the 305 having low-lying lesions requiring abdominoperineal resection, survival in the treated group was 46.9% compared with 34.3% in controls. Although suggestive of a treatment benefit, neither is considered statistically significant.

Histological positive lymph nodes were found in 41.2% of the control group and in only 27.8% of the patients receiving radiotherapy. Literature review shows this observation to be consistent in all reported trials. Review of all patients who died during the study shows a consistently lower death rate from cancer in the radiotherapy group. Interval survival data indicate that the treatment benefit only becomes evident during the fourth and fifth years of observation.

Currently we are conducting a randomized trial using 3,150 rad during a three-week preoperative period. Approximately 200 patients have been entered. No increase in operative morbidity or mortality has been observed in those receiving preoperative treatment. Review of resected specimens continues to substantiate previous observation that preoperative radiation reduces the number of positive lymph nodes.

APPENDIX

PRINCIPAL INVESTIGATORS

Dr. Dan Smith
Albuquerque, NM

Dr. Decio Rangel
Boston, MA

Dr. James McElhinney
Bronx, NY

Dr. Harry H. LeVeen
Brooklyn, NY

Dr. Thomas W. Shields
Chicago, IL

Dr. Darryl J. Sutorius
Cincinnati, OH

Dr. Jerry S. Wolkoff
Cleveland, OH

Dr. R. W. Postlethwait
Durham, NC

Dr. Nae K. Cheung
East Orange, NJ

Dr. Herbert Greenlee
Hines, IL

Dr. Gene Guinn
Houston, TX

Dr. Nelson Gurll
Iowa City, IA

Dr. J. Harold Conn
Jackson, MS

Dr. Robert Boudet
Kansas City, MO

Dr. Raymond Read
Little Rock, AR

Dr. George L. Juler
Long Beach, CA

Dr. Charles Frey
Martinez, CA

Dr. Joseph McCaughan
Memphis, TN

Dr. Edward Humphrey
Minneapolis, MN

Dr. Ernest Rosato
Philadelphia, PA

Dr. Felicien M. Steichen
Pittsburgh, PA

Dr. Jose H. Amadeo
San Juan, PR

Dr. Robert C. Donaldson
St Louis, MO

Dr. Lloyd S. Rogers
Syracuse, NY

Dr. Gale L. Mendeloff
Wood, WI

Dr. George A. Higgins
Washington, DC

REFERENCES

1. Buroker, T.; Nigro, N.; Correa, J.; Vaitkevicius, V.K.; Samson, M.; and Considine, B. (1976). Combination preoperative radiation and chemotherapy in adenocarcinoma of the rectum. *Dis Colon Rectum,* **19:**660–63.
2. Gerard, A.; and Wassif, S.B. Personal communications.

3. Higgins, G.A.; Conn, H.; Jordan, P.H.; Humphrey, E.W.; Roswit, B.; and Keehn, R.J. (1975). Preoperative radiotherapy for colorectal cancer. *Ann Surg,* **181:**624–31.

4. Kligerman, M.M.; Urdaneta, N.; Knowlton, A.; Vidone, R.; Hartman, P.V.; and Vera, R. (1972). Preoperative irradiation of rectosigmoid carcinoma including its regional lymph nodes. *Am J Roentgenol Radium Ther Nucl Med,* **114:**498–503.

5. Quan, S.H.; and Stearns, M.W., Jr. (1960). The effect of preoperative roentgen therapy upon the 10 and 5 year results of the surgical treatment of cancer of the rectum. *Surg Gynecol Obstet,* **111:**507.

6. Ruff, C.C.; Dockerty, M.B.; Fricke, R.E.; and Waugh, J.M. (1961). Preoperative radiation therapy for adenocarcinoma of rectum and rectosigmoid. *Surg Gynecol Obstet,* **112:**715–23.

7. Stearns, M.W.; Deddish, M.R.; Quan, S.H.; and Leaming, R.H. (1974). Preoperative roentgen therapy for cancer of the rectum and rectosigmoid. *Surg Gynecol Obstet,* **138:**584–86.

8. Stevens, K.R., Jr.; and Allen, C.V. (1976). Preoperative radiotherapy for adenocarcinoma of the rectosigmoid. *Cancer,* **37:**2866.

9. Wassif, S.B. (1974). A pilot study of a new regime of combined therapy for the radical treatment of marginally operable rectal (or colo-rectal) cancer. *Eur J Cancer,* **10:**615–19.

CHAPTER
18

Preoperative Radiotherapy in Rectal Cancer

Maus W. Stearns, Jr.

Chief, Rectum and Colon Service
Memorial Sloan-Kettering Cancer Center
New York, New York, U.S.A.

THE BEST ADJECTIVE to describe our experience at Memorial Sloan-Kettering Cancer Center with preoperative x-ray therapy in rectal cancer is frustration.

Dr. George Binkley, who started our specialized Rectal Service in the 1930s, had initially tried to treat cancer of the rectum by external radiation and intralumenal radium applicator. It was not many years before he gave up this attempt and concentrated on surgery. However, because he had had some radiation "cures" and had observed considerable regression in many tumors, he continued to use radiation therapy preoperatively in many patients. After World War II, with the advances in surgical physiology, antibiotics, anesthesia, and the enthusiasm of youth, we wore Dr. Binkley down and concentrated on an extended surgical attack. Our first disillusionment came when we reviewed our efforts with our extended surgical attack on rectal cancer of combining extended abdominal pelvic lymphadenectomy with surgical resection. We found we had not improved survival significantly but had increased the morbidity, particularly through urinary complications. We then decided the future was in adjuvant therapy, and so we reviewed among other things Dr. Binkley's considerable experience with preoperative radiation therapy.

To summarize this experience from 1939–1951,[1] we found a slightly, but not significantly, higher survival rate of those having resections who had had preoperative radiotherapy (Table I). This therapy had been given with 250 kV units, 450 roentgens in air per exposure, with tumor doses calculated not over 2,000 roentgens, although with recent interest in equivalent biologic effect it may have been higher. We reviewed a number of parameters: age (Table II), sex (Table III), grade of tumor (Table IV), none of which showed any differences. However, in those with regional nodal metastases the survival was significantly higher when preoperative radiotherapy had been given (Table V). Thus the determinate survival was 27% in 200 patients without radiation and 43% in 195 with radiotherapy preoperatively.

Since this was as good as we had achieved with the addition of abdominopelvic lym-

TABLE I
Five-Year Survival

	Total patients	Five-year survivors	Five-year survival rate (%)
Total series	1786	505	28.5
Operated upon	1276	479	37.4
No X ray	549	225	41.0
With X ray	727	254	35.0
Resected	971	479	49.0
No X ray	473	225	47.5
With X ray	498	254	51.0

TABLE II
Survival and Age

Age, years	No. of patients	Five-year survival rate (%)
Under 40		
No X ray	28	43
With X ray	36	70
40 to 49		
No X-ray	75	62
With X ray	99	55
50 to 59		
No X ray	133	52
With X ray	152	48
60 to 69		
No X ray	138	49
With X ray	151	53
Over 70		
No X ray	42	33
With X ray	38	37

TABLE III
Survival and Sex

	No. of patients	Five-year survival rate (%)
Males		
No X ray	302	48
With X ray	380	40
Females		
No X ray	169	53
With X ray	188	56

TABLE IV
Survival and Grade of Tumor

Grade of tumor	No. of patients	Five-year survival rate (%)
I		
No X ray	7	73
With X ray	8	75
II		
No X ray	232	57
With X ray	238	61
III		
No X ray	101	43
With X ray	178	47
IV		
No X ray	6	17
With X ray	6	33

phodenectomy without the associated morbility, we resumed the practice of preoperative radiation therapy in 1957. However, we were persuaded that there should be a control series. Since this was before the days of "informed consent," and since these were primarily patients seen in private offices, a simple method of randomization was agreed to which would allow us to advise the patient as to the indicated treatment when we initially saw and examined them. We used the patient's birthdate as a basis, and, although it is not as sophisticated as other methods, it was a practical way to meet the problem at the time. A defect later became apparent when we reviewed the series: there was a great disproportion of treated and control patients in the area above 11 cm. We discussed the problem, and it became apparent that we had not defined the rectum adequately, and so some investigators had not included this area in their randomization.

TABLE V
Survival and Dukes' Classification

Dukes' classification	No. of patients	Incidence in series (%)	Liver metastasis	Indeter-minate	Five-year survivors	Overall five-year survival (%)	Determinate five-year survival (%)
A							
No X ray	96	21	0	8	69	72	79
With X ray	103	23	2	15	75	73	85
B							
No X ray	145	33	0	12	92	63	70
With X ray	161	35	2	12	104	64	72
C							
No X ray	201	46	19	10	46	23	27
With X ray	195	43	13	14	72	37	43

TABLE VI
Preop X ray

	Overall	
	No X ray	Plus X ray
Total number patients	414	376
Indeterminate	44	57
Five-yr. survivors	242	215
Five-yr. survival		
Overall	58%	57%
Determinate	65%	67%

TABLE VII
Preop X ray Location

	No X ray	Plus X ray
Below 6 cm		
Determinate patients	62	70
Five-yr. survival	62%	56%
6–10 cm		
Determinate patients	114	170
Five-yr. survival	59%	66%
11–16 cm		
Determinate patients	184	76
Five-yr. survival	70%	68%

TABLE VIII
Preoperative X ray and Nodal Metastases

	No X ray	Plus X ray
Negative nodes		
Total No.	262	245
Indeterminate	31	36
Five-year survivors	182	164
Five-year survival overall	68%	67%
Five-year survival determinate	78%	79%
Positive nodes		
Total No.	152	131
Indeterminate	13	21
Incidence	37%	35%
Five-year survivors	63	49
Five-year survivals overall	41%	37%
Five-year survivals determinate	45%	44.5%

TABLE IX
APR

	No X ray	Plus X ray
Total	90	139
POD	0	6
Indeterminate-total	10	22
Five-yr. survivors	45	70
Ca. after five years	3	8
Five-year survival		
Overall	50%	50%
Determinate	55%	60%
NEC	53%	53%

We continued the randomized series from 1960 through 1967. In 1973, when we were able to evaluate the series, we met with more frustration.[2] We could not show that we had accomplished any improvement with our 11-year efforts. The overall survival in the control and treated patients was identical (Table VI), as it was regardless of the location (Table VII) and whether or not regional nodal metastases were present (Table VIII). What we did find, however, was that whereas in the early series the determinate five-year survival was only 27% in those having surgery alone, and 43% in those who had additional preoperative radiation, in the later series both the control and the treated patients had a 45% five-year survival. This suggested to us that in the early series we had improved our surgical efforts by preoperative X-ray therapy, whereas in the later group we had improved our surgical efforts so that radiation did not add anything demonstrable.

In view of the results reported by the Veterans Administration[3] on the value of preoperative X-ray therapy in those patients having treatment by abdominoperineal resection, we considered this group (Table IX). The results following that operation again showed no difference between those treated and those in the control group.

One analysis may be of interest, particularly in view of the Veterans Administration experience, and that has to do with sex difference (Table X). In the control group males showed poorer survival than women, the usual observation in studies of colon and rectal cancer, whereas in the treated group men and women showed similar survival rates, indicating, that the relative survival of men was improved.

TABLE X
Preop X ray—Sex

	No X ray		Plus X ray	
	Men	Women	Men	Women
Determinate patients	192	178	186	133
Five-yr. survivors	114	128	126	87
Determinate				
Five-yr. survival	59%	72%	68%	65%

TABLE XI
Incidence Nodal Metastases

	Total patients	Number nodal metastatses	Incidence
1939–1951			
No XRT	323	141	43%
Plus XRT	447	188	42%
1957–1967			
No XRT	414	152	37%
Plus XRT	376	131	35%

Finally, in view of the suggestion that there is a lower incidence of regional nodal metastases in those treated by preoperative x-ray therapy, we compared the incidence of nodal metastases in both of our series in which the patients had received about 2,000 rad tumor dose (Table XI). There is no difference in incidence.

In conclusion, we have been convinced that, in our patients treated by five or six surgeons performing similar surgical resection, two radiation therapists delivering similar radiation therapy, and the same pathologists examining the resected specimens, we could not demonstrate any increased survival attributable to routine use of preoperative radiation. At the present time preoperative therapy is indicated for patients with borderline operable lesions, specifically those which are partially fixed or deeply infiltrating into adjacent tissues.

REFERENCES

1. Stearns, M. W., Jr.; Deddish, M. R.; and Quan, S. H. Q. (1959). Preoperative roentgen therapy for cancer of the rectum. *Surg Gynecol Obstet,* **109:**225–29.
2. Stearns, M. W., Jr.; Deddish, M. R.; Quan, S. H. Q.; and Leaming, R. H. (1974). Preoperative roentgen therapy for cancer of the rectum and rectosigmoid. *Surg Gynecol Obstet,* **138:**584–86.
3. Higgins, G. A., Jr.; Conn, J. H.; Jordan, D. H., Jr.; Humphrey, E. W.; Roswit, B.; and Keehr, R. J. (1975). Preoperative radiotherapy for colorectal cancer. *Ann Surg* **181:**624–30.

The Clinical Relevance of Histopathologic Classification in Non-Hodgkin's Lymphoma

Steven E. Come

Division of Medical Oncology

Sidney Farber Cancer Institute

and

Beth Israel Hospital

Harvard Medical School

Boston, Massachusetts

George P. Canellos

Chief of Medicine

Sidney Farber Cancer Institute

Harvard Medical School

Boston, Massachusetts

INTRODUCTION

HISTOPATHOLOGIC SUBCLASSIFICATIONS of the malignant lymphomas and the definition of their relationship to leukemias and to other disorders of lymph nodes have been subjects of controversy and confusion since the presentation of Hodgkin's classic paper in 1832.[1] While the observations of Sternberg,[2] Reed,[3] and others[4,5] established Hodgkin's disease as a histopathologic entity by the early 1900s, characterization of the diverse disorders which comprise the non-Hodgkin's lymphomas has evolved more slowly. Follicular lymphomas were described by Brill in 1925[6] and Symmers in 1927.[7] Reticulum cell sarcomas of bone[8] and lymph node[9] were reported within the next five years. However, the division of non-Hodgkin's lymphomas into small cell lymphosarcoma, giant follicular lymphosarcoma, and reticulum cell sarcoma did not achieve clinical significance until the exhaustive review by Rosenberg[10] thirty years later. In 1956, Rappaport, Winter, and Hicks,[11] recognizing the lack of homogeneity of follicular lymphomas, proposed a new classification. This scheme, modified in 1966,[12] has provided the structure for a decade of productive clinical research on non-Hodgkin's lymphoma which promises to parallel the somewhat earlier therapeutic successes in Hodgkin's disease.

Simultaneously with this, advances in membrane biology led to the concept that lymphomas are neoplastic disorders of the lymphocyte at various levels of maturity. Techniques initially developed to identify the immunologic origin and function of normal lymphocytes have recently been applied to lymphoreticular malignancies.[13,14,15] This biologic characterization of lymphomas may provide a functional supplement to—and perhaps eventually replace—pure morphologic classification.

MORPHOLOGIC CHARACTERIZATION: THE RAPPAPORT CLASSIFICATION

In the Rappaport classification,[12] non-Hodgkin's lymphomas are stratified based on the pattern of tumor growth within the node and the cytologic features of the lymphoma cells. The pattern of growth, which can be accurately assessed only by inspection of multiple thin sections from an involved lymph node or spleen, may be nodular (follicular), simulating normal germinal centers, or, lacking this, considered diffuse. The cytologic analysis considers cell and nuclear size, nuclear configuration, chromatin pattern, and the degree of homogeneity of the malignant cells, using these characteristics to assign the tumor to one of five categories (Table I).

The prognostic accuracy of this morphologic approach to the classification of non-Hodgkin's lymphomas has been confirmed by the results of large clinical studies at Stanford,[16,17] the National Cancer Institute,[18] and elsewhere.[19,20] Each of these analyses has revealed a survival advantage for nodular as compared to diffuse tumors in general, with the exception of diffuse, well-differentiated lymphocytic lymphoma, which has a relatively indolent course and no nodular counterpart. Further, within a common pattern of growth, differences in prognosis can be related to cytology.

The Rappaport classification derives additional clinical relevance from the meticulously collected staging and natural history data from these same centers.[16,21] This information has established a relatively homogeneous clinical picture for each Rappaport subtype, with appreciable differences between subtypes. For example, nodular poorly differentiated lymphocytic lymphomas are usually disseminated at presentation with bone marrow and liver involvement in approximately $\frac{1}{2}$ of cases.[21] Conversely, diffuse histiocytic lymphomas are more likely localized and uncommonly involve the liver and marrow at presentation.[21] Although the total survival of patients with nodular poorly differentiated lymphocytic

TABLE I
Rappaport Classification (1966)

Pattern of growth	Nodular or diffuse
Cytology	Lymphocytic, well differentiated
	Lymphocytic, poorly differentiated
	Mixed cell, lymphocytic and histiocytic
	Histiocytic
	Undifferentiated

lymphoma who achieve complete remission is long, the median duration of complete remission—and hence the relapse-free survival—is short.[22] In contrast, the majority of complete remissions in patients with diffuse histiocytic lymphomas are long lasting, and the total survival in this histologic subtype is closely parallel to relapse-free survival.[22] Thus, assignment of a lymphoma to a Rappaport subtype confers certain clinical expectations, which may influence the staging and treatment. Therefore, the Rappaport classification has relevance not only to prognosis but also to the prospective management of the lymphoma patient.

Recent clinicopathologic and biologic observations create a need to update and modify Rappaport's 20-year-old proposal. For completeness, several newly-described entities must be added. Burkitt's lymphoma, first described in 1958,[23] has, at least in its African form, emerged as a specific clinical and immunologic disorder which can be pathologically separated from other undifferentiated lymphomas through the use of special techniques.[24] Lymphoblastic lymphoma, previously regarded as a tumor presenting in the mediastinum of adolescents,[25,26,27,28] is now recognized in adults, including the elderly, and found to have protean presentations.[29,30] Despite two cytologic forms[29]—convoluted and nonconvoluted—these cases share a common differentiation marker, terminal deoxynucleotidyl transferase, and a predilection for rapid conversion to an acute leukemia.[29,30,31] The distinctive clinicopathologic features and the poor response to conventional treatment necessitate the segregation of this disease from the diffuse poorly differentiated lymphocytic or undifferentiated categories in which it has been included.[29,32] Though its precise definition remains controversial,[11] "immunoblastic" sarcoma represents a third potential addition to the Rappaport scheme. Rappaport himself reserves this nomenclature for "lymphomas which are composed of large lymphoid cells with plasmacytoid features, and which arise in a pre-existing immunoproliferative process. . . ."[32] Mycosis fungoides, clinicopathologically recognized for years, has also recently been awarded a position in the non-Hodgkin's lymphoma family.

Not clarified in Rappaport's original or 1966 proposal is the classification of tumors which display evidence of nodular and diffuse growth in the initial biopsy material. A recent examination of this problem at Stanford[39] reveals that any degree of nodularity in lymphocytic or mixed lymphomas carries a favorable prognosis. Conversely, areas of diffuse involvement in nodular histiocytic tumors would confer a poorer prognosis. If reproducible, these clinical observations may provide guidelines for the pathologic classification of these previously ambiguous cases.

The term *histiocytic lymphoma*, like its predecessor, *reticulum cell sarcoma*, is a semantic and biologic inaccuracy for the majority of cases in this category. Studies of membrane surface markers[34,35] and histochemical characteristics[35] demonstrate that these morphologically similar tumors are primarily composed of functionally diverse transformed lymphocytes and only rarely of true histiocytes. Dorfman[36] has proposed replacing *histiocytic* with *large lymphoid*, reserving the former label for true histiocytic tumors. Similarly, the category of diffuse poorly differentiated lymphocytic lymphoma encompasses a range of syndromes that are heterogenous in cell of origin, clinical course, and response to treatment.

These additions, clarifications, and semantic corrections could be easily implemented and have been largely accepted by Rappaport.[32] However, the accuracy with which pure morphologic classification can be reproduced has been challenged and remains a major potential limitation of this approach. Correct interpretation of growth pattern, as judged by members of the Lymphoma Pathology Panel and Repository (LPPR),[37] was established in 95% of cases by pathologists at the University of Chicago Conference.[38] In a more recent report from the Southwest Oncology Group, pathologists from participating institutions achieved 91% agreement with the LPPR in identifying nodularity, but recognized diffuse growth in only 80% of lesions so considered by the LPPR.[39]

Cytologic subclassification appears to be less reproducible than assessment of pattern of growth. At the Chicago Conference, agreement with the LPPR was best for histiocytic and well-differentiated lymphocytic lymphomas, but occurred only in 74% and 72% of cases respectively. Poorly differentiated and mixed lymphomas were correctly identified in 64% and 69% of cases. In the Southwest Group study, agreement with the LPPR ranged from 61% for histiocytic lymphoma to 49% for poorly differentiated lymphocytic tumors. These studies emphasize the need for pathologic review of cases entered in major trials to maximize the interpretability of the results. Further, because of the frequent dependence of treatment on the Rappaport classification, they create some anxiety about the present management of non-Hodgkin's lymphoma in noninvestigational settings.

BIOLOGIC CHARACTERIZATIONS OF NON-HODGKIN'S LYMPHOMA

Considerable evidence suggests that lymphocytes can be divided into two functional groups.[40,41] One population is thymus dependent for differentiation (T cells), and the second is thymus independent and differentiates in a bursa equivalent (B cells). These B and T lymphocytes, as well as mononuclear phagocytes, can be distinguished by differences in membrane surface markers. B cells characteristically have surface immunoglobulin, a receptor for the Fc portion of the immunoglobulin molecule, and most have receptors for the third component of complement (C3).[14] Mononuclear phagocytic cells have a receptor for C3 but also have receptors for cytophilic antibody not present on B lymphocytes.[14] T cells, which have none of these membrane receptors, can be identified by their spontaneous formation of rosettes with sheep erythrocytes (E rosettes) or by the use of an anti-T lymphocyte antiserum.[14] Analyses of membrane receptors have primarily employed cell suspensions prepared from peripheral blood or mechanically disrupted tissue. More recently, techniques to detect receptors for C3 and for cytophilic antibody have been adapted for use in frozen sections of unfixed tissue.[42] When these methods are applied to normal lymph nodes, B cells are found predominantly in the germinal centers (follicles) and in the medullary cords, with T cells populating the paracortical regions. Mononuclear phagocytic cells are most abundant in the subcapsular and medullary sinuses but are also seen in paracortical regions and in reactive germinal centers.[14]

Both cell-suspension and frozen-section techniques have been used to study non-Hodgkin's lymphomas.[14] Nodular lymphomas of all cytologic subtypes display B cell properties, reflecting the putative germinal center origin of these tumors. Diffuse well-differentiated lymphocytic lymphomas have also invariably been typed as B-cell malignancies. The cells in these lesions are conceptually related to the lymphocytes differentiating towards plasma cells that are found in the normal medullary cords, the nonfollicular B-cell region of the lymph node. The postulated nonfollicular origin of this tumor may explain the observation that well-differentiated lymphocytic lymphomas rarely, if ever, display a true nodular growth pattern. Although the B cells of nodular lymphomas have densely staining surface immunoglobulins, usually IgM kappa or lambda light chains, and prominent C3 receptors, those of diffuse well-differentiated lymphocytic lymphomas have faintly staining surface immunogobulin and inconspicuous C3 receptors, similar to the cells of chronic lymphatic leukemia. Thus, two subpopulations of B cells are apparently discernible, with C3 receptors marking germinal center derivation. This finding parallels studies of normal lymphocytes, which reveal a reduction in C3 receptors as differentiation towards an immunoglobulin-producing cell proceeds.[43] Although Burkitt's lymphoma is recognized as a diffuse stem cell lymphoma, the membrane receptors are those of follicular B cells.[44] This concept is supported by the rare observation of selective germinal center involvement in this tumor.[14]

Lymphocytic lymphomas of intermediate differentiation fall cytologically between the cells of nodular poorly differentiated lymphocytic lymphoma and those of diffuse well-differentiated lymphocytic lymphoma. Surface studies of these tumors reveal that they are immunotypically intermediate as well, theoretically consistent with derivation from follicular cuff cells at the interface between the germinal center and the medullary cord.[35,45]

Surface receptor studies of diffuse lymphomas other than well-differentiated lymphocytic and Burkitt's tumor reveal heterogeneity in each morphologic subtype. Although many cases of diffuse poorly differentiated lymphocytic lymphoma have B-cell markers like their nodular counterparts, some forms are classified as T cell and others exhibit neither B- nor T-cell surface properties (*null cell*).[14] Similarly, B- and T-cell diffuse mixed lymphomas have been described.[14] Marker characterization of diffuse histiocytic lymphomas demonstrate that the majority of these tumors are transformed B lymphocytes rather than the reticulum cells or histiocytes that they resemble morphologically. Approximately $\frac{1}{4}$ of these tumors can be classified as null cell, while a small proportion are found to have either T-cell properties or to be composed of true phagocytic histiocytes.[35,46]

Lymphoblastic lymphoma, a relatively new term, defines a homogeneous clinical entity, which may have either convoluted or nonconvoluted lymphoid cells and displays considerable variability in surface markers in the small number of patients studied. The convoluted cell cases consistently form E rosettes that are characteristic of T cells. Some of these cases have also been shown to possess C3 receptors.[30,35,47] Although the C3 receptor has been considered a B-cell marker, it has also recently been demonstrated on fetal thymocytes.[48] The nonconvoluted cell cases may also have C3 receptors alone or in combination with E rosette formation, E rosette formation alone, or no markers.[35,47] At present the surface properties of these tumors are thought to reflect various defects in the differentiation of primitive T cells.[47] In most cases tested, cells from mycosis fungoides and the Sezary's syndrome form E rosettes; thus, these disorders are classified as T-cell malignancies.[14]

Assay for activity of terminal deoxynucleotidyl transferase (TdT), a unique DNA-polymerizing enzyme, has enabled further biologic characterization of the non-Hodgkin's lymphomas. This enzyme has been demonstrated in the lymphoid elements of the thymus[49]

and in the blast cells from some cases of acute lymphoblastic leukemia[50] and chronic myelogenous leukemia in blast crisis.[51] No detectable activity of TdT is present in mature or
phytohemagglutinin-stimulated lymphocytes.[51] When TdT is assáyed in non-Hodgkin's
lymphomas, activity is uniformly detected in lymphoblastic lymphoma, regardless of
cytologic or surface properties. Low but significant activity has also been observed in one
diffuse histiocytic lymphoma characterized as null cell by the absence of membrane receptors.[31] No enzyme activity has been measured in the cells from cases of Sezary's syndrome. Thus, analogous to the subpopulations of B cells described previously, subsets of
T cells can be distinguished. TdT activity and C3 receptors, with or without E rosette formation, appear to mark primitive or immature T cells, while mature or peripheral T cells
are detected by E rosette formation and/or anti-T lymphocyte antiserum in the absence
of TdT activity and C3 receptors. No TdT activity has been recorded in B-cell non-Hodgkin's lymphomas.[31]

Several cyto- and histochemical markers have been demonstrated to complement surface
receptor analysis in non-Hodgkin's lymphoma. Immunoperoxidase staining of fixed-tissue
sections can be used to detect cytoplasmic immunoglobulin in B cells and muramidase in
mononuclear phagocytic cells.[15] Alkaline phosphatase activity has been described in follicular and follicular-cuff B cells.[52] Acid phosphatase and B-glucuronidase staining has been
reported in a spectrum of T-cell disorders ranging from lymphoblastic lymphoma to Sezary's
syndrome and T-cell chronic lymphatic leukemia.[35] Alpha-naphthylacetate esterase pos-
itivity provides a marker for true histiocytes.[15]

NEWER CLASSIFICATIONS OF NON-HODGKIN'S LYMPHOMAS

The application of these immunologic and biochemical techniques has enhanced the
understanding of normal lymphocyte biology and of the relationship between normal and
malignant cells. These recently established concepts have spawned new classifications of
non-Hodgkin's lymphomas which combine cytologic and immunologic analysis seeking
improved biologic accuracy and reproducibility.

THE LUKES-COLLINS CLASSIFICATION

This scheme, originally proposed in 1973,[53] views non-Hodgkin's lymphomas as disorders
of the B- and T-cell systems. Fundamental to this approach is the recognition of a close
parallel between the cells of the normal lymphoid follicle and those observed in nodular
lymphomas.[54] The normal follicular center is postulated to be the site of B-cell transformation based on the resemblance of follicular center cells (FCC) to lymphocytes transformed
in vitro.[55] Theoretically, a small, round B lymphocyte at the follicular cuff, following an-
tigenic stimulation, undergoes a sequential metamorphosis in the follicular center to a small
cleaved FCC, a large cleaved FCC, a small noncleaved FCC, and ultimately to a large,
noncleaved FCC. The noncleaved FCCs are considered to be the proliferative elements
of the follicular center and give rise to plasma cell precursors. Noncleaved FCCs may mi-

TABLE II
Lukes-Collins Classification (1973)

B-cell types
    Small lymphocyte (CLL)
    Plasmacytoid lymphocyte
    Follicular center cell (FCC) types
        small cleaved
        large cleaved
        small noncleaved
        large noncleaved
    B-cell immunoblastic sarcoma
    Hairy cell leukemia

T-cell types
    Small lymphocyte
    Mycosis fungoides and Sezary's syndrome
    Convoluted lymphocyte
    T-cell immunoblastic sarcoma
    Lennert's lymphoma

U-cell (undefined) types

Histiocytic type

Unclassifiable

grate to interfollicular regions where, as B-cell immunoblasts, they may continue to produce plasma cell precursors. Normal T cells are postulated to undergo transformation in non-follicular areas of the node.

According to Lukes and Collins, the small, round B lymphocyte, each of the FCCs, the B-cell immunoblast, and the plasmacytoid lymphocyte can be recognized morphologically. B-cell lymphomas reflect malignant proliferation of one or another of these normal elements (Table II). Lymphomas that arise from different stages of T-cell transformation can also be identified morphologically by these authors.

In practice, Lukes and Collins rely on morphology to determine immunotype and cytologic subgroup, which are then correlated with independently performed surface marker and cytochemical characterizations. Their experience with 384 cases of non-Hodgkin's lymphoma and lymphatic leukemias reveals concordance of morphologic impression and laboratory data for B- and T-cell tumor.[55] In this series, 67% of cases were classified as B-cell malignancies, one-half of these being of FCC origin. Fifteen percent of cases were considered to be T-cell lymphomas with tumors of convoluted lymphocytes and immunoblastic sarcomas the most frequent designations. Seventeen percent of cases, all clinically acute lymphoblastic leukemia of childhood, were undefinable (U cell) by their immunologic and cytochemical methods. True histiocytic tumors, comprising 1% of the study, were identified by alpha naphthyl butyrate staining.

The relationship of the Lukes-Collins scheme to that of Rappaport is illustrated by a recent clinicopathologic study in which 202 cases of non-Hodgkin's lymphomas were retrospectively reclassified using the morphologic guidelines of each system.[56] In a group of 111 nodular lymphomas, 98 were poorly differentiated lymphocytic by the Rappaport scheme. All but two of these corresponded to the Lukes-Collins small, cleaved FCC subgroup. Thus, for the overwhelming majority of nodular lymphomas, the Lukes-Collins classification offers only a change in name. In a diffuse growth pattern, 11 of 12 Rappaport poorly differentiated lymphocytic lymphomas could also be classified as Lukes-Collins small, cleaved FCC tumors. Of the 54 diffuse lymphomas classified as Rappaport *histiocytic* or large-cell tumor,[36] 42 (78%) of these corresponded to the Lukes-Collins large, noncleaved FCC subtype. Half of the 12 cases assigned other Lukes-Collins designations were considered B-cell immunoblastic sarcomas, a subtype whose separation from the large, noncleaved FCC subgroup is both difficult and of uncertain clinical relevance. Of the 18 Rappaport malignant lymphoma-lymphoblastic cases, 10 were Lukes-Collins convoluted cell tumors. The other eight, which had blastic cytologic features but no convolutions, did not fit any existing Lukes-Collins category. Therefore, for the diffuse lymphomas, each major Rappaport group—poorly differentiated lymphocytic, "histiocytic," and lymphoblastic—corresponded with only one Lukes-Collins subtype in 63 of 84 cases (75%). A single modification of the Lukes-Collins system, which would expand the convoluted lymphoma category to include tumors of lymphoblasts without convolutions, would increase this one-to-one correspondence to 85%. On clinical grounds such a modification appears justifiable based on Nathwani's findings.[29]

Hence, the Lukes-Collins classification largely replaces one homogeneous Rappaport class with a new homogeneous class of more modern nomenclature. Although the Lukes-Collins approach does subdivide the Rappaport histiocytic category, the heterogeneity of which has been increasingly recognized,[35] it substitutes its own ambiguity in the U-cell subgroup, which may contain at least three different Rappaport types—histiocytic, lymphoblastic, and undifferentiated.

Since extensive correlations of clinical data with Lukes-Collins subtypes have yet to be compiled, the relevance of this classification with respect to prognosis and natural history is not yet established. Although, as in the Rappaport system, cytology appears to be prognostically important in this classification, the significance of growth pattern is controversial. Lukes has stated that, at least for small, cleaved FCC tumors, there is no survival advantage for a follicular versus a diffuse pattern of growth.[32] Butler, however, applying the Lukes-Collins classification to a series of previously studied cases, did demonstrate a clear survival advantage for lesions with follicular pattern.[57] Similarly, Nathwani observed a statistically significant difference in median survival between follicular and diffuse FCC tumors.[56]

The promise in the Lukes-Collins classification lies in its yet-to-be confirmed biologic accuracy and its potential to detect functional differrences among morphologically similar lesions. However, the assumption that classification based on function or immunotype has more clinical relevance than one based on pattern of growth has not been sustantiated. Several disadvantages of this classification are apparent. The accuracy of morphologic diagnosis, perhaps the Achilles heel of the Rappaport system, seems unlikely to be improved by the Lukes-Collins scheme. The diagnosis of immunoblastic sarcomas, particularly of the T-cell type, and of true histiocytic tumors has proven difficult for the most experienced pathologist.[32,56] No morphologic guidelines have been established for the U-cell category.

Further, special techniques, not presently widely utilized, are required for the fixation, sectioning, and staining of tissue.[15,32] Excessive cell loss in preparation of specimens from large, noncleaved FCC tumors—exactly the subtype in which the Lukes-Collins classification might be most useful—is encountered in Lukes' own hands. Finally, the performance and interpretation of immunologic and cytochemical procedures remains fraught with error.[15] The development of specific, accurate anti-B and anti-T cell antisera may ameliorate this latter problem and permit reassignment of cases which are currently relegated to the U-cell category.

THE KIEL CLASSIFICATION

The Kiel classification, proposed by Gerard-Marchant[58] and Lennert,[59] like that of Lukes and Collins, recognizes that the majority of non-Hodgkin's lymphomas are of FCC origin and are the counterparts of normal germinal center cells. In this system (Table III), tumors are stratified by grade of malignancy rather than immunotype and are further subdivided based on cytology. The suffix -cytic is used to convey low and -blastic, high grades of malignancy. The centrocyte corresponds to one or both of Lukes' cleaved FCCs, while the centroblast is a noncleaved FCC. Immunoblastic in this classification would be applied to all tumors considered histiocytic by Rappaport, except those that can be demonstrated to be of follicular center origin. Thus, the Kiel immunoblastic lymphoma does not correspond to the immunoblastic sarcoma of Lukes, which is more narrowly defined and applies to only 10%[56] of Rappaport histiocytic lymphomas.

Like the Rappaport and the Lukes-Collins classifications, the Kiel system relates prognosis to cytology, in particular the proportion of centroblasts in centroblastic-centrocytic tumors. Further, as in the Lukes-Collins classification, the impact of growth pattern on prognosis is discounted.

TABLE III
Kiel Classification (1974)

Low-grade malignancy
    Malignant lymphoma (ML)—lymphocytic (CLL and others)
    ML—lymphoplasmacytoid (immunocytic)
    ML—centrocytic
    ML—centroblastic-centrocytic

High-grade malignancy
    ML—centroblastic
    ML—lymphoblastic
    —Burkitt's type
    —convoluted-cell type
    —other
    ML—Immunoblastic

Though achieving a measure of acceptance in Europe,[60] the utility of the Kiel classification is hampered by its cumbersome terminology and its ambiguous cytologic criteria. While its functional concepts, which are similar to those proposed by Lukes and Collins, may prove to be biologically correct, there is little to suggest that it is more easily reproducible or more clinically relevant than the recently proposed modifications of the Rappaport classification.[32,36] Like the Lukes-Collins classification, the Kiel system seems in direct conflict with the accumulated clinical data, which reflects the prognostic importance of growth pattern.

CONCLUSIONS

As the non-Hodgkin's lymphomas are pathologically, clinically, and biologically diverse, the therapeutic and investigative necessity to subclassify these tumors seems clear. The classification based purely on morphology, proposed by Rappaport twenty years ago and periodically modified, has proven clinical relevance. The reproducibility of this semi-quantitative analysis is not optimal, although error can be minimized by careful adherence to Rappaport's criteria.[61] The use of this classification by a number of centers in the United States has allowed for the development of a common "language," which has contributed to the rapid progress in the understanding of the impact of therapy on the various subtypes of the non-Hodgkin's lymphomas. Developments in lymphobiology have been quickly translated into new functional classifications schemes, although the underlying concepts as yet lack substantiation. Based on biology at a time when biology is rapidly changing, these classifications, in addition, appear more difficult to apply than the Rappaport approach. The available clinical correlations using these newer systems are still limited, so their clinical relevance, as well, remains uncertain. Both the Lukes-Collins and the Kiel classifications fail to acknowledge the significance of growth pattern which, well supported by clinical data, emerges as the major prognostic determinant in the Rappaport scheme.

The Rappaport classification is in need of additions and modifications in nomenclature to comply with newer concepts that can be universally accepted.[32] With these changes, it remains a durable approach that should enjoy continued clinical use. The further refinement and application of immunologic and cytochemical techniques to the non-Hodgkin's lymphomas in the research setting should ultimately provide the information from which classification of these tumors can be revised in a manner that is sound clinically and biologically.

REFERENCES

1. Hodgkin, T. (1832). On some morbid appearances of the absorbent glands and spleen. *Med-Chir Trans*, 17:68–114.
2. Sternberg, C. (1902). Über eine eigenartige unter dem bilde der pseudoleukamie verlaufende tuberculose des lymphatischen apparates. *Z Heilk*, 19:133–96.
3. Reed, D. M. (1902). On the pathologic changes in Hodgkin's disease, with special reference to its relation to tuberculosis. *Johns Hopkins Hosp Rep*, 10:133–96.

4. Langhans, T. (1872). Das maligne lymphosarkom (Pseudolenkämie). *Virchow's Arch Pathol Anat,* **54:** 509–37.

5. Greenfield, W. S. (1878). Specimens illustrative of the pathology of lymphadenoma and leucocythemia. *Trans Pathol Soc London,* **29:**272–304.

6. Brill, N. E.; Baehr, G.; and Rosenthal, N. (1925). Generalized giant lymph follicle of lymph nodes and spleen. A hitherto undescribed type. *J Am Med Assoc,* **84:**668–71.

7. Symmers, D. (1927). Follicular lymphadenopathy with splenomegaly. A newly recognized disease of the lymphatic system. *Arch Pathol Lab Med,* **3:**816–20.

8. Oberling, C. (1928). Les réticulosar comes et les réticuloendotheliosarcomes de la moelle osseuse (sarcomes d'Ewing). *Bull Assoc Franç-étude du cancer,* **17:**256–96.

9. Roulet, F. (1930). Das primäre rotothelsaskom der lymphknsten. Virchows *Arch Pathol Anat,* **277:**15–47.

10. Rosenberg, S. A.; Diamond, H. D.; Jaslowitz, B. et al. (1961). Lymphosarcoma: A review of 1269 cases. *Medicine,* **40:**31–84.

11. Rappaport, H.; Winter, W. J.; Hicks, E. B. (1956). Follicular lymphoma. A re-evaluation of its position in the scheme of malignant lymphomas, based on a survey of 253 cases. *Cancer,* **9:**792–821.

12. Rappaport, H. (1966). Tumors of the hematopoietic system. *Atlas of Tumor Pathology,* Section III, Fascicle 8, Armed Forces Institute of Pathology, Washington, D.C.

13. Siegal, F. P.; Filippa, D. A.; and Koziner, B. (1978). Surface markers in leukemias and lymphomas. *Am J Pathol,* **90:**457–60.

14. Braylan, R. C.; Jaffe, E. S.; and Berard, C. W. (1975). Malignant lymphomas: Current classification and new observations. In *Pathology Annual 1975* S. C. Sommers (Ed.), Appleton-Century-Crofts, New York, 213–70.

15. Lukes, R. J.; Taylor, C. R.; Chir, M. B. et al. (1978). A morphologic and immunologic surface marker study of 299 cases of non-Hodgkin's lymphomas and related leukemias. *Am J Pathol,* **90:**461–86.

16. Jones, S. E.; Fuks, Z.; Bull, M. et al. (1973). Non-Hodgkin's lymphomas. IV. Clinicopathologic correlation in 405 cases. *Cancer,* **31:**806–23.

17. Portlock, C. S., and Rosenberg, S. A. (1977). Chemotherapy of the non-Hodgkin's lymphomas: The Stanford experience. *Cancer Treat Rep,* **61:**1049–55.

18. Schein, P. S.; Chabner, B. A.; Canellos, G. P. et al. (1974). Potential for prolonged disease-free survival following combination chemotherapy of non-Hodgkin's lymphoma. *Blood,* **43:**181–89.

19. Brown, T. C.; Peters, M. V.; Bergsagel, D. E. et al. (1974). A retrospective analysis of the clinical results in relation to the Rappaport histologic classification. *Br J Cancer (Suppl. II),* **31:**208–216.

20. Bloomfield, C. D.; Goldman, A.; Dick, F. et al. (1974). Multivariate analysis of prognostic factors in the non-Hodgkin's lymphomas. *Cancer,* **33:**870–79.

21. Chabner, B. A.; Johnson, R. E.; DeVita, V. T. et al. (1977). Sequential staging in non-Hodgkin's lymphoma. *Cancer Treat Rep,* **61:**893–997.

22. Anderson, T.; Bender, R. A.; Fisher, R. I. et al. (1977). Combination chemotherapy in non-Hodgkin's lymphoma: Results of long-term follow-up. *Cancer Treat Rep,* **61:**1057–66.

23. Burkitt, D. (1958). A sarcoma involving the jaws in African children. *Br J Surg,* **46:**218–23.

24. Berard, C. W.; O'Connor, G. T.; Thomas, L. B. et al. (Eds.) (1969). Histopathological definition of Burkitt's tumor. *Bull WHO,* **40:**601–607.

25. Jones, B., and Klingberg, W. G. (1963). Lymphosarcoma in children. A report of 43 cases and review of the literature. *J Pediatr,* **63:**11–20.

26. Kaplan, J.; Mastrangelo R.; and Peterson, W. D., Jr. (1974). Childhood lymphoblastic lymphoma, a cancer of thymus-derived lymphocytes. *Cancer Res,* **34:**521–25.

27. Pinkel, D.; Johnson, W.; and Aur, R. J. A. (1975). Non-Hodgkin's lymphoma in children. *Br J Cancer,* (Suppl. II) **31:**298–323.

28. Sen, L., and Borella, L. (1975). Clinical importance of lymphoblasts with T markers in childhood acute leukemic. *N Engl J Med,* **292:**828–31.

29. Nathwani, B. N.; Kim, H.; and Rappaport, H. (1976). Malignant lymphoma, lymphoblastic. *Cancer,* **38:** 964–83.

30. Rosen, P. J.; Feinstein, D. I.; Pattengale, P. K. et al. (1978). Convoluted lymphocytic lymphoma in adults. A clinicopathologic entity. *Ann Intern Med,* **89:**319–24.

31. Donlon, J. A.; Jaffe, E. S.; and Braylan, R. C. (1977). Terminal deoxynucleotidyl transferase activity in malignant lymphomas. *N Engl J Med*, **297**:461–64.

32. Berard, C. W., Chairman (1977). Discussion II: Round table discussion of histopathologic classification. *Cancer Treat Rep*, **61**:1037–48.

33. Warnke, R. A.; Kim, H.; Fuks, Z. et al. (1977). The coexistence of nodular and diffuse patterns in nodular non-Hodgkin's lymphoma significance and clinicopathologic correlation. *Cancer*, **40**:1229–33.

34. Brouet, J. C.; Preud'homme, J. L.; Flandrin, G. et al. (1976). Membrane markers in "histiocytic" lymphomas (reticulum cell sarcoma). *J Natl Cancer Inst*, **56**:631–33.

35. Jaffe, E. S.; Braylan, R. C.; Nanba, K. et al. (1977). Functional markers: a new perspective on malignant lymphomas. *Cancer Treat Rep*, **61**:953–62.

36. Dorfman, R. F. (1977). Pathology of the non-Hodgkin's lymphomas: New classifications. *Cancer Treat Rep*, **61**:945–51.

37. DeVita, V. T.; Rappaport, H.; and Frei, E., III (1968). Announcement of formation of the Lymphoma Task Force and Pathology Reference Center. *Cancer*, **22**:1087–88.

38. Berard, C. W., and Dorfman, R. F. (1974). "Histopathology of Malignant Lymphomas." In *Clinics in Hematology*, S. A. Rosenberg (Ed.), W. B. Saunders, Philadelphia, 3, 39–76.

39. Jones, S. E.; Butler, J. J.; Byrne, G. E. et al. (1977). Histopathologic review of lymphoma cases from the Southwest Oncology Group. *Cancer* **39**:1071–76.

40. Raff, M. C. (1970). Two distinct populations of peripheral lymphocytes in mice distinguishable by immunoflourescence. *Immunology*, **19**:637–50.

41. Raff, M. C. (1973). T and B lymphocytes and immune responses. *Nature*, **242**:19–23.

42. Jaffe, E. S.; Shevach, E. M.; Sussman, E. H. et al. (1975). Membrane receptor sites for the identification of lymphoreticular cells in benign and malignant conditions. *Br J Cancer* (Suppl. II), **31**:107–120.

43. Bianco, C.; Patrick, R.; and Nussenzweig, V. (1970). A population of lymphocytes bearing a membrane receptor for antigen-antibody-complement complexes. I. Separation and characterization. *J Exp Med*, **132**:702–720.

44. Mann, R. B.; Jaffe, E. S.; Braylan, R. C. et al. (1976). Non-endemic Burkitt's lymphoma: A B cell tumor related to germinal centers. *N Engl J Med*, **295**:685–91.

45. Jaffe, E. S.; Shevach, E. M.; Frank, M. M. et al. (1974). Nodular lymphoma: Evidence for origin from follicular B lymphocytes. *N Engl J Med*, **290**:813–19.

46. Bloomfield, C. D.; Kersey, J. H.; Brunning, R. D. et al. (1977). Prognostic significance of lymphocytic surface markers and histology in adult non-Hodgkin's lymphoma. *Cancer Treat Rep*, **61**:963–70.

47. Jaffe, E. S.; Braylan, R. C.; Frank, M. M. et al. (1976). Heterogeneity of immunologic markers and surface morphology in childhood lymphoblastic lymphoma. *Blood*, **48**:213–22.

48. Gatien, J. G.; Schneeberger, E. E.; and Merler, E. (1975). Analysis of human thymocyte subpopulations using discontinuous gradients of albumin: Precursor lymphocytes in human thymus. *Eur J Immunol*, **5**:312–17.

49. Chang, L. M. S. (1971). Development of terminal deoxynucleotidyl transferase activity in embryonic calf thymus gland. *Biochem Biophys Res Commun*, **44**:124–31.

50. McCaffrey, R.; Harrison, T. A.; Parkman, R. et al. (1975). Terminal deoxynucleotidyl transferase in human leukemic cells and in normal human thymocytes. *N Engl J Med*, **292**:775–80.

51. Sarin, P. S.; Anderson, P. N.; and Gallo, R. C. (1976). Terminal deoxynucleotidyl transferase activities in human blood leukocytes and lymphoblast cell lines: High levels in lymphoblast cell lines and blast cells of some patients with chronic myelogenous leukemia in acute phase. *Blood* **47**:11–20.

52. Nanba, K.; Jaffe, E. S.; Braylan, R. C. et al. (1977). Alkaline phosphatase-positive malignant lymphoma. A subtype of B cell lymphomas. *Am J Clin Pathol*, **68**:535–42.

53. Lukes, R. J., and Collins, R. D. (1973). New observations on follicular lymphoma. In *Malignant Disease of the Hematopoietic System*, GANN Monograph on Cancer Research No. 15, K. Akazaki, H. Rappaport, C. W. Berard, J. M. Bennett, and E. Ishikawa (Eds.), University of Tokyo Press, Tokyo, 209–215.

54. Glick, A. D., and Leech, J. H.; Waldron, J. A. et al. (1975). Malignant lymphomas of follicular center cell origin in man. II. Ultrastructural and cytochemical studies. *J Natl Cancer Inst*, **54**:23–36.

55. Lukes, R. J., and Collins, R. D. (1977). Lukes-Collins classification and its significance. *Cancer Treat Rep*, **61**:971–79.

56. Nathwani, B. N.; Kim, H.; Rappaport, H. et al. (1978). Non-Hodgkin's lymphomas. A clinicopathologic study comparing two classifications. *Cancer*, **41**:303–325.

57. Butler, J. J.; Stryker, J. A.; and Shullenberger, C. C. (1975). A clinicopathological study of stage I and II non-Hodgkin's lymphomata using the Lukes-Collins classification. *Br J Cancer* (Suppl. II), **31**:208–216.

58. Gerard-Marchant, R.; Hamlin, I.; Lennert, K. et al. (1974). Classification of non-Hodgkin's lymphomas. *Lancet* **2**:406–8.

59. Lennert, K.; Mohri, N.; Stein, H. et al. (1975). The histopathology of malignant lymphoma. *Br J Haematol*, (Suppl.), **31**:193–203.

60. Bartels, H.; Bremer, K.; Brittinger, G. et al. (Sept. 1976). Clinical significance of the Kiel classification of non-Hodgkin's lymphomas (NHL). In *Proceedings of the 16th International Congress of Hematology*, Kyoto, Japan, 60.

61. Byrne, G. E.; Jr. (1977). Rappaport classification of non-Hodgkin's lymphoma: Histologic features and clinical significance. *Cancer Treat Rep*, **61**:935–44.

Clinical Relevance of the Kiel Classification of Non-Hodgkin Lymphomas: Preliminary Results of a Prospective Multicentric Study*

G. Brittinger

Hämatologische Abteilung der Medizinischen Universitätsklinik Essen
Essen, West Germany

U. Schmalhorst, H. Bartels, H. Brücher, H. Common, E. Dühmke, H. H. Fülle, U. Gunzer, D. Huhn, E. König, K. Lennert, H. Leopold, P. Meusers, L. Nowicki, H. Pralle, A. Stacher, and H. Theml

Kiel Lymphoma Study Group

INTRODUCTION

IN RECENT YEARS, the rapidly expanding knowledge of the physiology and pathophysiology of the immune system has led to attempts to classify the non-Hodgkin lymphomas according to immunological and functional instead of morphological criteria alone. Among such new classifications considered to be scientifically more accurate than the "classical" European and the Rappaport classifications,[19] both based on pure morphology, is the Kiel classification, which was proposed in 1974 by Lennert and a group of other European pathologists[8,13] and which has gained increasing interest in Europe as well as in the United States.

This classification (Table I) differentiates two main groups of non-Hodgkin lymphomas, those of low-grade and of high-grade malignancy. The lymphomas of low-grade malignancy are subdivided into a lymphocytic type, comprising the chronic lymphocytic leukemia (CLL) and other rarer subentities such as the Sézary syndrome, the mycosis fungoides, and

* Supported by the Deutsche Krebshilfe e.V., Bonn, Germany

TABLE I
Kiel Classification of Non-Hodgkin Lymphomas (1974)

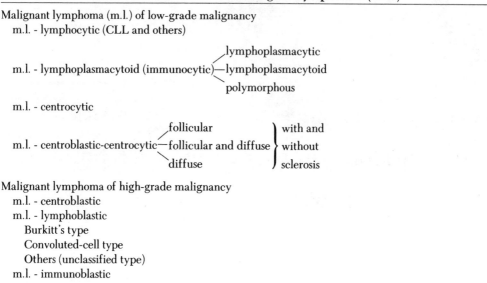

Malignant lymphoma (m.l.) of low-grade malignancy
   m.l. - lymphocytic (CLL and others)

   m.l. - lymphoplasmacytoid (immunocytic)—lymphoplasmacytic / lymphoplasmacytoid \ polymorphous

   m.l. - centrocytic

   m.l. - centroblastic-centrocytic—follicular / follicular and diffuse \ diffuse } with and without sclerosis

Malignant lymphoma of high-grade malignancy
   m.l. - centroblastic
   m.l. - lymphoblastic
     Burkitt's type
     Convoluted-cell type
     Others (unclassified type)
   m.l. - immunoblastic

the prolymphocytic leukemia, and into a lymphoplasmacytoid or immunocytic type that has three histopathologic subtypes: the lymphoplasmacytic, the lymphoplasmacytoid, and the polymorphous type. Waldenström's macroglobulinemia is part of this lymphoma entity. The histopathologic criteria of low-grade malignancy are also fulfilled by the centrocytic and the centroblastic-centrocytic lymphomas, which are considered to be neoplasias originating from germinal center cells. The centrocytic lymphoma might be related to the diffuse, poorly differentiated lymphocytic lymphoma of the Rappaport classification.[13,15] The centroblastic-centrocytic lymphoma has a follicular, a follicular and diffuse, and a diffuse variant, all manifesting with or without sclerosis, and is presumably identical with a high proportion of the nodular lymphomas according to Rappaport.[13,14] Malignant lymphomas of high-grade malignancy are classified as centroblastic (another neoplasia of the germinal center cells), as lymphoblastic, and as immunoblastic. The lymphoblastic lymphomas are histologically subdivided into a Burkitt's (B-cell) type, a convoluted (T-cell) type, and an unclassified type, in which the majority is non-T/non-B-cell neoplasias. The immunoblastic lymphoma seems to correspond, at least in part, to the diffuse histiocytic lymphoma of the Rappaport classification.[13,20]

    Clinical use of a new histopathologic classification is based on a satisfactory correlation between the various histologic entities and more or less specific clinical and especially prognostic features as shown to be true for the Rappaport classification by many studies performed during the past decade.[7,10,11,22] Since the clinical relevance of the Kiel classification had not yet been tested, the Kiel Lymphoma Study Group, which comprises several clinicians at different institutions in West Germany and Austria, first initiated the retrospective analysis of 405 patients with non-Hodgkin lymphomas diagnosed according to this classification schema.[1,2,3,24] The data obtained from this investigation demonstrated the prognostic relevance of the histologic subdivision into lymphomas of low-grade and high-grade malignancy and, in addition, differences of survival between entities belonging to the group of malignant lymphomas of low-grade malignancy. Furthermore, clinical features characteristic of certain lymphoma entities could become evident. However, since in these patients the diagnostic and therapeutic procedures, as well as the follow-up, had not been performed according to a single protocol, data regarding certain clinical features such as initial stage distribution were not always available. Therefore, in October 1975 the Kiel Lymphoma Study Group started a prospective multicentric study.[4]

PROTOCOL AND RESULTS

Principles of the Protocol

The diagnostic protocol[4] requires staging of all consecutive, previously untreated patients admitted to the various institutions according to a modification by Musshoff[17] of the Ann Arbor classification.[5] In the presumably localized stages I and II, extended field irradiation is performed, whereas patients with the more advanced stages III and IV receive chemotherapy and additional radiotherapy, applied at least to involved regions. An exception, differing from the general therapeutic protocol, is the very radiosensitive centroblastic-centrocytic lymphoma;[6,18] it is treated in stage III patients with total lymphoid irradiation only. Furthermore, in children and young adults with all stages of lymphoblastic lymphoma, which apparently has a high tendency to generalize early during the course of the disease[12,16] chemotherapy plus radiotherapy of the involved regions plus CNS prophylaxis are given. In adult patients over 30 years of age with this disease the chemotherapeutic regimen is identical with that used in other lymphomas of high-grade malignancy.

The data given in this paper are primarily based on an interim evaluation of this prospective study, which is still in progress, and, in addition, on results of the retrospective study.

Distribution of Histologic Subtypes

The distribution of the histologic subtypes among 384 patients registered for the prospective study (Table II) shows a strong predominance of non-Hodgkin lymphomas of low-grade malignancy, the leading entities being the lymphoplasmacytoid and the lymphocytic lymphomas. The centroblastic-centrocytic lymphoma represents only 15.1% if the total population is considered, and no more than 18% if the CLL is omitted (this is not included in the non-Hodgkin lymphomas in the Rappaport classification). Assuming that the centroblastic-centrocytic lymphoma is identical with the majority of the nodular lymphomas according to Rappaport and that in the United States about 25–30% of all non-Hodgkin lymphomas are of the nodular poorly differentiated lymphocytic variety,[39] the low incidence of the centroblastic-centrocytic lymphoma is surprising and favors the

TABLE II
Distribution of Histologic Subtypes, Prospective Study[a]

	No. of patients	%
M.l. of low-grade malignancy	277	72.1
Lymphocytic		
CLL	62	16.1
Others	17	4.4
Lymphoplasmacytoid (LP)	93	24.2
Centrocytic (CC)	38	9.9
Centroblastic-centrocytic (CB-CC)	58	15.1
Borderline cases (CLL/LP, CB-CC/LP; CC/CB-CC)	8	2.1
Unclassifiable	1	0.3
M.l. of high-grade malignancy	94	24.5
Centroblastic (CB)	25	6.5
Lymphoblastic (LB)	16	4.2
Immunoblastic (IB)	33	8.6
Unclassifiable	20	5.2
Lymphogranulomatosis X	13	3.4
	384	100.0

[a] m.l. = malignant lymphoma. CLL = chronic lymphocytic leukemia.

hypothesis that the incidence of certain non-Hodgkin lymphoma entities shows geographic differences.[15]

Clinical Features Common to the Groups of Non-Hodgkin Lymphomas of Low-Grade and High-Grade Malignancy

At the time of interim evaluation (February 1978) data of 269 out of the 384 patients registered for the study were available.

Age distribution: As shown on Figure 1, non-Hodgkin lymphomas of low-grade malignancy are very rarely observed before the forth decade of life, reaching their peak incidence between 60 and 70 years of age. In contrast, lymphomas of high-grade malignancy, especially of the lymphoblastic type, also arise in children and young adults, with a subsequent age distribution analogous to that of the lymphomas of low-grade malignancy.

Prognosis: In an attempt to investigate the clinical significance of the histopathologic differentiation into low-grade and high-grade malignant lymphomas, actuarial survival of patients belonging to these groups was compared.

Figure 2 demonstrates that the 314 patients of the retrospective study with lymphomas of low-grade malignancy manifested a 50% survival probability of 72 months, which is significantly superior to the 9 months found in the 91 patients with lymphomas of high-grade malignancy.

In the prospective study, after a follow-up period of only 26 months, patients with high-grade malignant lymphomas showed a probability of survival of only 0.34 as compared to the patients with lymphomas of low-grade malignancy having a probability of survival of 0.66 (Fig. 3). This significant prognostic difference between the two major groups of

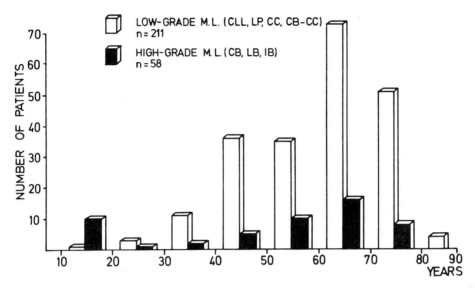

Fig. 1. Age distribution of non-Hodgkin lymphoma patients; prospective study. For abbreviations see Table II.

non-Hodgkin lymphomas is analogous to the well-known longer survival of patients with nodular lymphomas, in comparison to patients with diffuse lymphomas of the Rappaport classification.[10,11,12]

Rapidity of lymph node enlargement, constitutional (B) symptoms, initial bone marrow involvement, and blood lymphocytosis: As for survival, patients with low-grade and high-grade malignant lymphomas also showed differences with regard to the rapidity of lymph node enlargement as evidenced from patient's history (Table III). Whereas 62% of the patients with a subtype of the malignant lymphomas of high-grade malignancy noticed a rapid growth of their lymph nodes within less than three months, in the majority of the patients with malignant lymphomas of low-grade malignancy the lymph nodes en-

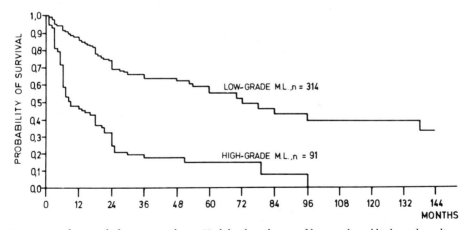

Fig. 2. Actuarial survival of patients with non-Hodgkin lymphomas of low-grade and high-grade malignancy; retrospective study. M.L. = malignant lymphoma.

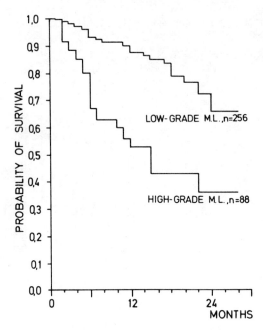

Fig. 3. Actuarial survival of patients with non-Hodgkin lymphomas of low-grade and high-grade malignancy; prospective study. M.L. = malignant lymphoma.

larged only slowly. These results can be interpreted as reflecting a higher growth fraction of the malignant lymphomas of high-grade malignancy as compared to the low-grade malignant subtypes.

These data are in line with recent observations by Silvestrini et al.[23] showing a labeling index after incubation in vitro of lymph node cells with ^{3}H-thymidine, which gradually increased from the different low-grade to the high-grade malignant lymphoma entities. Unlike rapidity of lymph node enlargement, frequency of constitutional (B) symptoms as defined by the Ann Arbor classification[5] on the whole did not parallel the degree of lymphoma malignancy, even though some differences between single entities could be

TABLE III
Clinical and Hematological Data of Patients with Non-Hodgkin Lymphomas of Low-Grade and High-Grade Malignancy; Prospective Study

	Malignant lymphomas	
	of low-grade malignancy	of high-grade malignancy
Rapid lymph node enlargement (<3 months)	32/174 (18%)	23/37 (62%)
Constitutional (B) symptoms (1–3 symptoms)	95/200 (48%)	24/48 (50%)
Initial bone marrow involvement	153/200 (77%)	17/45 (38%)
Initial blood lymphocytosis (>4,000/μl)	107/199 (54%)	4/48 (8%)

distinguished (Table III). Thus, in contrast to Hodgkin's disease, the prognostic relevance of the presence or absence of B symptoms seems to be doubtful, as previously pointed out by the Stanford group.[21]

Initial bone marrow involvement was found to be much more frequent in patients with low-grade malignant lymphomas than in patients with high-grade malignant entities (Table III).

In the group of patients with low-grade malignant lymphomas there was a decreasing incidence of bone marrow involvement from 100% in CLL, 87% in lymphoplasmacytoid, and 76% in centrocytic, to only 45% in centroblastic-centrocytic lymphoma. Although mean incidence of bone marrow involvement was lower in high-grade malignant lymphomas, clear-cut differences could be demonstrated between the centroblastic and immunoblastic lymphomas (24 and 31%, respectively) and the lymphoblastic lymphomas (67%). There are preliminary data suggesting that in lymphoma entities with a low incidence of bone marrow involvement there is a considerable proportion of patients exhibiting localized disease at diagnosis.

Initial blood lymphocytosis of more than 4,000 cells per μl was less frequently observed in both low-grade and high-grade malignant lymphoma patients than initial bone marrow involvement (Table III). So far, it has not been established whether or not bone marrow involvement is always accompanied by the appearance of atypical lymphocytes in the peripheral blood even though total lymphocyte count is normal.

Clinical Features of Single Lymphoma Entities

Chronic lymphocytic leukemia and lymphoplasmacytoid lymphoma: Considering CLL and lymphoplasmacytoid lymphoma (Table IV), age and sex distribution are apparently similar; however, initial bone marrow involvement and blood lymphocytosis are less frequent in lymphoplasmacytoid lymphoma than in CLL. Presence of a monoclonal serum immunglobulin of the IgM or another class is highly indicative of a lymphoplasmacytoid lymphoma, but three-quarters of the patients are lacking this alteration. The data show that in many patients differential diagnosis between these two lymphoma entities is difficult

TABLE IV
Clinical and Hematological Data of Patients with Chronic Lymphocytic Leukemia and Lymphoplasmacytoid Lymphoma; Prospective Study

Chronic lymphocytic leukemia: $n = 47$	
Age: Median: 64	Range: 35–84 years
Sex: ♂ : ♀	1.3:1
Initial bone marrow involvement:	100%
Initial blood lymphocytosis (>4,000/μl):	96%
Monoclonal serum gammopathy:	2%
Malignant lymphoma, lymphoplasmacytoid: $n = 86$	
Age: Median: 66	Range: 28–80 years
Sex: ♂ : ♀	1.1:1
Initial bone marrow involvement:	87%
Initial blood lymphocytosis (>4,000/μl):	65%
Monoclonal serum gammopathy:	26%

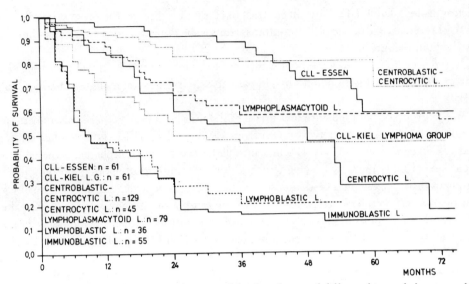

Fig. 4. Actuarial survival of patients with non-Hodgkin lymphomas of different histopathology according to the Kiel classification; retrospective study.

or even impossible using clinical and hematological criteria alone and must be reached by histopathology and immunology.

Differential diagnosis seems necessary, however, since data of the retrospective study (Fig. 4) and results of the prospective study (Fig. 5) have shown that patients with a lymphoplasmacytoid lymphoma have a shorter survival than patients with CLL. It must be emphasized, however, that the relatively poor prognosis of a group of patients with CLL of the retrospective study called the CLL-Kiel Lymphoma Study Group can be attributed to the fact that at that time lymph node biopsy was not done in all consecutive patients with CLL but only in selected cases, so that an accumulation of patients with aggressive or advanced disease can be assumed.

Centrocytic and centroblastic-centrocytic lymphoma: The clinical and hematological features of the two low-grade malignant lymphomas originating from germinal center cells are different with respect to several parameters (Table V). Median age of patients with a centrocytic lymphoma is almost one decade higher than that of patients with a centroblastic-centrocytic lymphoma. There is a strong preponderance of males in centrocytic and of females in centroblastic-centrocytic lymphoma. Initial bone marrow involvement is more frequent in centrocytic than in centroblastic-centrocytic lymphoma. Initial blood lymphocytosis is verified in only one-quarter of patients with centrocytic lymphoma and almost never in centroblastic-centrocytic lymphoma. Atypical lymphocytes such as centrocytes in centrocytic and centrocytes and/or centroblasts in centroblastic-centrocytic lymphoma, which in both diseases can be observed even at normal total lymphocyte counts, are seen more frequently in the centrocytic than in the centroblastic-centrocytic entity. The higher proliferative tendency of the centrocytic lymphoma is reflected by a rapid lymph node enlargement noticed by almost half of the patients as compared to only 16% of patients

TABLE V

Clinical and Hematological Data of Patients with Centrocytic and Centroblastic-Centrocytic Lymphoma; Prospective Study

Malignant lymphoma, centrocytic: $n = 25$	
Age: Median: 63	Range: 28–82 years
Sex: ♂ : ♀	3.1:1
Initial bone marrow involvement:	76%
Initial blood lymphocytosis ($>4,000/\mu l$):	24%
Atypical blood lymphocytes at diagnosis:	36%
Monoclonal serum gammapathy:	0%
Rapid lymph node enlargement (<3 months):	45%
Malignant lymphoma, centroblastic-centrocytic: $n = 42$	
Age: Median: 54	Range: 19–81 years
Sex: ♂ : ♀	0.4:1
Initial bone marrow involvement:	45%
Initial blood lymphocytosis ($>4,000/\mu l$):	2%
Atypical blood lymphocytes at diagnosis:	13%
Monoclonal serum gammapathy:	2%
Rapid lymph node enlargement (<3 months):	16%

with centroblastic-centrocytic lymphoma. A higher grade of malignancy of the centrocytic lymphoma is documented in the six years follow-up of the retrospective study (Fig. 4) by a shorter survival of patients with this disease than of patients with centroblastic-centrocytic lymphoma. Since the curve after 4.5 years approached that of patients with lymphoblastic and immunoblastic lymphomas with regard to prognosis, centrocytic lymphoma can be considered as an intermediate entity between typical low-grade and typical high-grade malignant lymphomas. This view is in keeping with the results obtained in vitro by Silvestrini et al.[23]

Centroblastic and immunoblastic lymphomas: The high-grade malignant centroblastic and immunoblastic lymphomas are characterized by very similar clinical and hematological parameters (Table VI). Median age of patients with these entities is between 60 and 70 years;

TABLE VI

Clinical and Hematological Data of Patients with Centroblastic and Immunoblastic Lymphoma; Prospective Study

Malignant lymphoma, centroblastic: $n = 24$	
Age: Median: 68	Range: 27–89 years
Sex: ♂ : ♀	0.8:1
Initial bone marrow involvement:	24%
Initial blood lymphocytosis ($>4,000/\mu l$)	0%
Initial blood lymphocytopenia ($<1,000/\mu l$):	17%
Malignant lymphoma, immunoblastic: $n = 18$	
Age: Median: 63	Range: 16–79 years
Sex: ♂ : ♀	0.8:1
Initial bone marrow involvement:	31%
Initial blood lymphocytosis ($>4,000/\mu l$):	6%
Initial blood lymphocytopenia ($<1,000/\mu l$):	22%

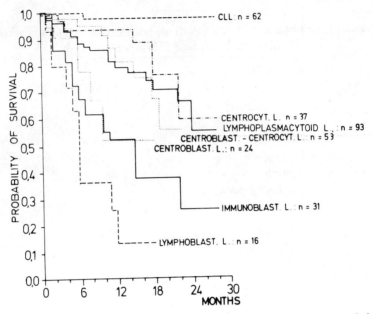

Fig. 5. Actuarial survival of patients with non-Hodgkin lymphomas of different histopathology according to the Kiel classification; prospective study.

sex distribution is almost balanced. Initial bone marrow involvement is seen in only one-quarter to one-third of patients and is only very rarely accompanied by blood lymphocytosis. Initial blood lymphocytopenia can be found in about 20% of patients.

Data available from the prospective study (Fig. 5) do not support the view that survival of patients with centroblastic lymphoma is different from that of patients with immunoblastic lymphoma. Thus, at the present time histopathologic differentiation between centroblastic and immunoblastic lymphoma seems to be of only minor clinical and prognostic relevance.

Lymphoblastic lymphoma: The lymphoblastic lymphoma is subdivided into three types: the convoluted-cell type, the Burkitt's type, and the unclassified type. It is observed in children and young adults as well as in older patients between 50 and 80 years of age. The convoluted-cell type and the Burkitt's type are most frequently seen between the first and second decade of life, whereas the unclassified type is equally distributed among all age groups (Fig. 6).

As shown on Table VII, all subtypes show a clear-cut predominance of males. At diagnosis, B symptoms, a mediastinal tumor, bone marrow involvement, blood lymphocytosis, and presence of atypical lymphocytes in the peripheral blood are most common in the convoluted-cell type and, at a lower rate, in the unclassified type. These symptoms and signs, however, have only rarely or not at all been noticed in patients with the Burkitt's type. Nevertheless, median survival of patients with all subtypes have not shown any differences so far, suggesting that the aforementioned clinical parameters might be of little or no prognostic value.

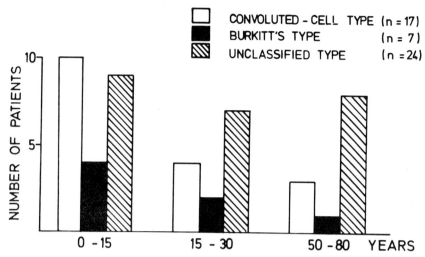

Fig. 6. Age distribution in lymphoblastic lymphoma; retrospective and prospective study.

CONCLUSION

The data of the retrospective study and the preliminary results of the prospective study of the Kiel Lymphoma Study Group demonstrate that there are clear-cut clinical, and especially prognostic, differences between the lymphomas of low-grade and high-grade malignancy. With regard to the various subentities of both groups, different types of results were obtained. In the lymphocytic lymphoma CLL and in the lymphoplasmacytoid lymphoma, clinical and hematological similarities were striking, but actuarial survival was different. Thus, in these cases histopathologic differentiation is necessary to allow appro-

TABLE VII
Clinical and Hematological Data of Patients with the Various Types of Lymphoblastic Lymphoma; Retrospective and Prospective Study

Malignant lymphoma, lymphoblastic: $n = 48$

Type	Convoluted-cell ($n = 17$)	Burkitt's ($n = 7$)	Unclassified ($n = 24$)
Sex: ♂ : ♀	1.8:1	2.5:1	2.4:1
Rapid lymph node enlargement (<3 months):	91%	67%	78%
B symptoms:	54%	17%	33%
Initial bone marrow involvement:	64%	0%	61%
Mediastinal tumor at diagnosis:	67%	14%	39%
Initial blood lymphocytosis (>4,000/μl):	40%	0%	11%
Atypical blood lymphocytes at diagnosis:	47%	0%	17%
Median survival (months):	8	8	8

priate clinical and prognostic judgement of the disease. In the centrocytic and centroblastic-centrocytic lymphomas clinical, hematological, and prognostic differences became evident, resulting in patterns relatively specific for each disease. Finally, in the centroblastic and the immunoblastic lymphomas, neither clinical and hematological nor prognostic differences could be found so far, suggesting that in these lymphoma entities histopathologic differentiation might be of minor relevance for the clinician.

The data available at the present time do not give appropriate information on several clinical aspects such as initial-stage distribution, frequency and localization of extranodal manifestations, mode of spread of the disease, and effectiveness of therapeutic regimens. It is expected that this information will come from the final evaluation of the prospective study. In order to compare the Kiel and Rappaport classifications from a clinical point of view, lymph-node biopsies from the patients of the prospective study will be reevaluated according to the Rappaport classification.

REFERENCES

1. Bremer, K.; Bartels, H.; Brittinger, G.; Burger, A.; Dühmke, E.; Gunzer, U.; König, E.; Stacher, A.; Theml, H.; and Waldner, R. (Kiel Lymphoma Group) (1977). Clinical significance of the Kiel classification of non-Hodgkin's lymphomas (NHL). In *Topics in Hematology*, Intern. Congress Series, No. 415, S. Seno, F. Takaku, and S. Irino (Eds.), Excerpta Medica, Amsterdam, 352–55.

2. Brittinger, G.; Bartels, H.; Bremer, K.; Dühmke, E.; Gunzer, U.; König, E.; and Stein, H. (Kieler Lymphomgruppe) (1976). Klinik der malignen Non-Hodgkin-Lymphome entsprechend der Kiel-Klassifikation: Centrocytisches Lymphom, centroblastisch-centrocytisches Lymphom, lymphoblastisches Lymphom, immunoblastisches Lymphom. In *Maligne Lymphome und monoklonale Gammopathien*, H. Löffler, (Ed.), *Hämatologie und Bluttransfusion*, Lehmann, München, 18:211–23.

3. Brittinger, G.; Bartels, H.; Bremer, K.; Burger, A.; Dühmke, E.; Gunzer, U.; König, E.; Stacher, A.; Stein, H.; Theml, H.; and Waldner, R. (Kieler Lymphomgruppe) (1977). Retrospektive Untersuchungen zur klinischen Bedeutung der Kiel-Klassifikation der malignen Non-Hodgkin-Lymphome. *Strahlentherapie*, 153:222–28.

4. Brittinger, G. (for the Kiel Lymphoma Study Group) (1978). Outline of a prospective multicentric study on the clinical significance of the Kiel classification of non-Hodgkin's lymphomas. In *Lymphoid Neoplasias: Clinical and Therapeutic Aspects*, G. Mathé, M. Seligmann, and M. Tubiana (Eds.), *Recent Results in Cancer Research*, Springer, Berlin-Heidelberg-New York 65:195–99.

5. Carbone, P.P.; Kaplan, H.S.; Musshoff, K.; Smithers, D.W.; and Tubiana, M. (1971). Report of the committee on Hodgkin's disease staging classification. *Cancer Res*, 31:1860–61.

6. Cox, J.D.; Koehl, R.H.; Turner, W.M.; and King, F.M. (1974). Irradiation in the local control of malignant lymphoreticular tumors (non-Hodgkin's malignant lymphoma). *Radiology*, 112:179–85.

7. DeVita, V.T. (1977). Summary of symposium. *Cancer Treat Rep*, 61:1223–27.

8. Gérard-Marchant, R.; Hamlin, I,; Lennert, K.; Rilke, F.; Stansfeld, A.G.; and van Unnik, J.A.M. (1974). Classification of non-Hodgkin's lymphomas. *Lancet* II:406–8.

9. Goffinet, D.R.; Warnke, R.; Dunnick, N.R.; Castellino, R.; Glatstein, E.; Nelsen, T.S.; Dorfman, R.F.; Rosenberg, S.A.; and Kaplan, H.S. (1977). Clinical and surgical (laparotomy) evaluation of patients with non-Hodgkin's lymphomas. *Cancer Treat Rep*, 61:981–92.

10. Jones, S.E.; Fuks, Z.; Bull, M.; Kadin, M.E.; Dorfman, R.F.; Kaplan, H.S.; Rosenberg, S.A.; and Kim, H. (1973). Non-Hodgkin's lymphomas. IV. Clinicopathologic correlation in 405 cases. *Cancer*, 31:806–23.

11. Jones, S.E. (1974). Clinical features and course of the non-Hodgkin's lymphomas. *Clin Haematol*, 3:131–60.

12. Landbeck, G.; Gaedicke, G.; Winkler, K.; and Stein, H. (1976). Besonderheiten der malignen Lymphome im Kindesalter. In *Maligne Lymphome und monoklonale Gammopathien*, H. Löffler (Ed.), *Hämatologie und Bluttransfusion*, Lehman, München, 18:225–35.

13. Lennert, K.; Mohri, N.; Stein, H.; and Kaiserling, E. (1975). The histopathology of malignant lymphoma. *Br J Haematol*, **31** (Suppl.):193–203.

14. Lennert, K. (1976). Klassifikation und Morphologie der Non-Hodgkin-Lymphome. In *Maligne Lymphome und monoklonale Gammopathien*, H. Löffler (Ed.), *Hämatologie und Bluttransfusion*, Lehmann, München, **18**:145–66.

15. Lennert, K. (Unpublished observation).

16. Murphy, S.B. (1977). The management of childhood non-Hodgkin's lymphoma. *Cancer Treat Rep*, **61**: 1161–73.

17. Musshoff, K., and Schmidt-Vollmer, H. (1975). Prognosis of non-Hodgkin's lymphomas with special emphasis on the staging classification. *Z Krebsforsch*, **83**:323–41.

18. Musshoff, K.; and Slanina, J. (1976). Maligne Systemerkrankungen. In *Strahlentherapie. Radiologische Onkologie*, E. Scherer (Ed.), Springer, Berlin-Heidelberg-New York, 705–88.

19. Rappaport, H. (1966). Tumors of the hematopoietic system. In *Atlas of Tumor Pathology*, sect. III, fasc. 8, Armed Forces Institute of Pathology, Washington, D.C., 91–156.

20. Rappaport, H. (1977). Roundtable discussion of histopathologic classification. *Cancer Treat Rep*, **61**: 1037–48.

21. Rosenberg, S.A.; Dorfman, R.F.; and Kaplan, H.S. (1975). A summary of the results of a review of 405 patients with non-Hodgkin's lymphoma at Stanford University. *Br J Cancer*, **31**, Suppl. II:168–73.

22. Rosenberg, S.A. (1977). Validity of the Ann Arbor staging classification for the non-Hodgkin's lymphomas. *Cancer Treat Rep*, **61**:1023–27.

23. Silvestrini, R.; Costa, A.; Daidone, M.G.; and Rilke, F. (1978). Prognostic significance of the labeling index in non-Hodgkin human malignant lymphomas. *Antibiot Chemother*, **24**:105–11.

24. Stacher, A.; Waldner, R.; and Theml, H. (Kieler Lymphomgruppe) (1976). Klinik der malignen Non-Hodgkin-Lymphome entsprechend der Kieler Klassifikation: Lymphoplasmozytoides Lymphom (LPL) und chronisch lymphatische Leukämie (CLL). In *Maligne Lymphome und monoklonale Gammopathien* H. Löffler (Ed.), *Hämatologie und Bluttransfusion*, Lehmann, München, **18**:199–209.

25. Stein, H. (1976). Klassifikation der malignen Non-Hodgkin-Lymphome aufgrund gemeinsamer morphologischer und immunologischer Merkmale zwischen normalen und neoplastischen lymphatischen Zellen. *Immunität und Infektion* **4**, 52–69, 95–109.

Management of Patients with Early Stages of Ovarian Carcinoma

Emmanuel van der Schueren, Dionisio Gonzalez, and Klaas Breur

Department of Radiotherapy
Wilhelmina Gasthuis
University of Amsterdam
Amsterdam-Oud-West
The Netherlands

INTRODUCTION

THE TREATMENT OF PATIENTS with ovarian carcinoma remains one of the more frustrating experiences in oncologic practice. The results have shown no improvement in the last decades,[17] and with an overall survival rate of about 30% it has become a more important cause of death than malignancies from cervix and corpus uteri combined.[1] This becomes even more puzzling when it is realized that the anti-tumor effect of surgery, radiotherapy, and chemotherapy in treating certain stages of this disease was demonstrated a long time ago.

Some explanation for the bad results can be found in the anatomical situation of the primary tumor. Malignant tumors of the ovary can reach fairly large volumes before they lead to signs or symptoms, which are usually vague and atypical. The situation of the ovaries in relation to the peritoneal cavity can result in tumor dissemination in an early stage of the disease. These two factors, easy dissemination and late symptoms, are responsible for the fact that about 70% of the patients presenting for first treatment have tumor spread outside the pelvis.[49]

However, even in the patient groups which were considered to have only disease confined to the pelvis at the time of diagnosis, results have been extremely disappointing. Patients in which the tumor involved only the ovaries (stage I) have had five-year survivals of about 60%, while in the group of patients with disease limited to the pelvis (stage II) only 40% are alive five years after treatment.[95,6]

The reasons for such poor results in apparently limited processes can be twofold: either the existing therapies are inefficient or they are used in a less than optimal way, part of the tumor extent being overlooked, resulting in a systematic undertreatment or nontreatment of certain tumor localizations. To check these two possibilities we shall first evaluate the normal tumor evolution and, second, estimate the efficacy of the known treatment modalities for the different stages of the tumor.

Histologically, ovarian tumors comprise a very heterogeneous group of tissues. The five tumor types which are grouped together by the FIGO[56] as epithelial tumors (serous, mucinous, endometrioid, mesonephric, and undifferentiated carcinoma) cover 80 to 90% of all ovarian tumors. We shall limit this discussion to these epithelial tumors.

Natural History of Ovarian Carcinoma

All known mechanisms of spread of malignant cells through the organism take place in the ovarian carcinoma:

1. direct invasion of surrounding tissues
2. seeding in a natural cavity (peritoneal)
3. lymphogenic metastases
4. hematogenic metastases
5. iatrogenic spread (spill during operation)

The most important and best recognized of these mechanisms of tumor spread are the peritoneal seeding and the direct invasion, as they are usually responsible for symptoms and the most common cause of death.

The other ways of tumor spread do occur, however; the lymphatic spread especially requires more extensive investigation to determine its exact role in the progression of this disease.

Direct invasion. The direct invasion of other tissues is the basis for the staging of limited disease (see Table I for FIGO classification) and will determine the local resectability of the tumors.

Stage I is limited to one (Ia) or two (Ib) ovaries, while stage II includes regional disease within the pelvis. Stage Ic is a separate category in which patients are included where macroscopic disease is stage I but where the presence of ascites suggest microscopic dissemination outside the pelvis.

It is noteworthy that a special category is made for patients with bilateral involvement of the ovaries (Ib). The occurrence of such tumor involvement of both the ovaries is around 10% for the mucinous and endometrioid carcinomas and even over 30% for the serous carcinomas, all in stage I. For higher stages of the disease, the incidence of bilateral involvement is more than twice these numbers.[67,88] This will have direct repercussions on the primary surgical treatment, requiring in nearly all the cases a bilateral oöphorectomy, even for limited processes. Bilateral tumor localization seems to carry a worse prognosis than unilateral involvement.[4]

In stage Ia a difference is made between processes which grow intracapsularly (Ia$_1$) and those with invasion of the capsule or with rupture of a tumor cyst during operation (Ia$_2$). Webb et al.[101] found a great difference in prognosis (98% vs. 68%) for these groups. This

TABLE I

F.I.G.O. Stagegroups for Primary Carcinoma of the Ovary (Used from 1/76)

Stage I	Growth limited to the ovaries.
Ia	Growth limited to one ovary; no ascites
	(1) No tumor on the external surface; capsule intact.
	(ii) Tumor present on the external surface or/and capsule ruptured.
Ib	Growth limited to both ovaries; no ascites
	(i) No tumor on the external surface; capsule intact.
	(ii) Tumor present on the external surface or/and capsule(s) ruptured.
Ic	Tumor either stage Ia or stage Ib, but with ascites[a] present or positive peritoneal washings.
Stage II	Growth involving one or both ovaries with pelvic extension.
IIa	Extension and/or metastases to the uterus and/or tubes.
IIb	Extension to other pelvic tissues.
IIc	Tumor either stage IIa or stage IIb, but with ascites[a] present or positive peritoneal washings.
Stage III	Growth involving one or both ovaries with intraperitoneal metastases outside the pelvis and/or positive retroperitoneal nodes. Tumor limited to the true pelvis with histologically proven malignant extension to small bowel or omentum.
Stage IV	Growth involving one or both ovaries with distant metastases. If pleural effusion is present there must be positive cytology to allot a case to stage IV. Parenchymal liver metastases equals stage IV.
Special category	Unexplored cases, thought to be ovarian carcinoma.

[a] Ascites is peritoneal effusion, which in the opinion of the surgeon is pathologic and/or clearly exceeds normal amounts.

could probably be explained by an increased probability of peritoneal seeding when the capsule is infiltrated or ruptured.

In stage II there seems to be an important difference between invasion of genitalia interna (IIa) or of other pelvic structures (IIb). Survival of patients with stage IIa is close to patients with stage I (60%), while a stage IIb carries a definitely worse prognosis (40%). This could be due to differences in biological characteristics, where invasion of tuba or uterus would be the expression of normal extension of tumor tissue to related tissues, while invasion of bladder or bowel could point to a more aggressively growing tumor. Also, in stage IIb a radical enbloc operation is usually not possible, so that chances for tumor spill are much larger than during an operation for a stage IIa.

Spread through the peritoneal cavity. As this is the most frequent cause of death,[10] this form of tumor spread is the best known and documented, although it appears that its extent is probably still very often underestimated. More than half of the ovarian tumor stages I and II appear to have tumor cells on the abdominal surface of the capsule,[36] and in the majority of patients malignant cells can be found in the peritoneal fluid or in peritoneal washings during laparotomy.[50]

The drainage mechanism of fluid from the peritoneal cavity has been known for a long time to the anatomists, but its implications seem to have been ignored by oncologists until very recently. The respiratory movements of the diaphragm function as a pumping mechanism with alternating increases and decreases of the pressure immediately below the diaphragm.[26,71] This results in a very rapid movement through the peritoneal cavity of any substance injected which is found in the diaphragm within a few minutes.[63,89] The fluid then passes through the diaphragm,[34] to the subpleural lymph nodes[16] and the retrosternal nodes.[15] This pathway makes it obvious that, although the whole peritoneal cavity is threatened by malignant cells in the peritoneal fluid, the first and greatest risk of implantation metastases would be in the diaphragm.

It was pointed out by Rutledge[87] that only one-third of all patients with pleural effusions have parenchymal lung metastases. This could be explained by the fact that these two localizations may be the result of two totally different ways of spread of the tumor. The pleural effusion would be due to direct spread of tumor cells from the peritoneal cavity to the subpleural lymph nodes, and the lung metastases could be due to hematogenic spread.

The role of the diaphragm as the most important station for peritoneal metastases was already suggested by Holm-Nielsen,[45] and Bergman[10] signalled in his autopsy series 50% of positive retrosternal lymph nodes. The need for the exploration of the diaphragm in the staging procedures of ovarian carcinoma was stressed by Bagley et al.[7] and by Feldman and Knapp.[31]

These diaphragmatic metastases possibly play a role in the pathogenesis of the ascites, which is frequently found in patients with ovarian carcinoma. Although it has been suggested[43] that ascites is due to increased production of peritoneal fluid, this has not been confirmed. On the contrary, it has often been observed that patients with extensive peritoneal metastases or peritonitis do not develop ascites. The normal capability for the resorption of peritoneal fluid appears to be very high, and it is unlikely that an increase of production could disturb this balance.[16,79]

Again it was Holm-Nielsen[45] who suggested that the development of ascites was probably due to blocking of the lymphatic channels by tumor cells. This hypothesis received new support from the experiments of Feldman et al.,[32] who demonstrated tumor localizations in the diaphragm and decreased resoprtion from the peritoneal cavity just before the development of ascites in mice. Also, the isotope clearance studies of Coates et al.,[15] point in this direction. They found that in patients with ascites due to liver cirrhosis there was a normal transit of particles from the abdomen to the mediastinum, while the movement was strongly reduced in patients with ascites due to ovarian carcinoma.

The implications of these data would be important in treatment decisions of those patients who were staged as Ic up to now. If the ascites found in these patients were indeed due to tumor infiltration of the diaphragm, then these cases could not be considered as "limited" anymore. The prognostic value of ascites in patients in whom the diaphragm was carefully evaluated will have to be redetermined

Lymph-node metastases. The lymphatic drainage of the ovary usually goes along with the ovarian vessels to the para-aortic nodes between the renal hilus and the bifurcatio aortae. In about half of the women an alternative way leads to the iliacal nodes, and very rarely there can be another channel along the ligamentum rotundum to the inguinal nodes.

The importance of tumor dissemination via lymphatic ways and its possible repercussion on the course of this disease and on the outcome of the treatment is unknown. Only recently has the routine use of lymphangiographies in some centers drawn attention to the relatively high incidence of lymph-node metastases. In the Stanford series,[36,41,74] an incidence of 22% positive lymphangiograms was found, and even in the patients with limited disease (stages I and II) positive nodes were found in 18% of the cases.

Other series[3,25,35,68] found radiological evidence of lymph-node metastases with frequencies ranging from 20 to 50% of all patients investigated. Knapp and Friedman[52] performed routine nodal biopsies in the lumbo-aortic region of 26 unselected patients with ovarian carcinoma stage I or II. In five cases (19%), tumor invasion of these nodes existed. It is noteworthy that the positive cases were all undifferentiated processes. It is very difficult to make an assessment of the incidence of lymph-node metastases in patients with early stages of ovarian carcinoma. Many studies do not separate their patients according to stage, and very often lymphangiography was performed on clinical indication, thus selecting a group of patients with higher chance of metastases. A reasonable estimate would be somewhere between 10 and 20%.[36,52,68] Undifferentiated tumors seem to be a group with a larger frequency of metastases[36,68] than would be expected from what is generally known about such types of processes.

Although the best-known lymphatic drainage is to the lumbo-aortic nodes, metastases are also found frequently in the iliacal and inguinal nodes.[3] This is probably due to the invasion of other pelvic structures, so that lymphogenic metastases follow the lymph drainage ways of these other organs, and also to possible modification of normal lymph flow after the invasion of nodes. Positive inguinal nodes thus were only found when the iliacal nodes were already invaded.

It is interesting to note that invasion of iliacal nodes alone, without metastases in the para-aortic region, was found in 25% of all patients with nodal metastases by Parker et al.,[74] and even in 54% by Musumeci et al.[68] These nodes would be covered by a routine pelvic irradiation field. The repercussions of lymph-node metastases on the natural history of this disease are unknown. One would expect them seriously to lessen the prognosis also, because, in analogy with other disease, they would lead to an increased incidence of hematogenic metastases. However, in the majority of patients treatment failures occur in the pelvis or the peritoneal cavity and only a small number die of distant metastases with control of the local tumor.[87] Lymph-node metastases do not seem to play a role in ascites formation either,[3] and isolated nodal recurrences as often seen in other gynecological malignancies are rare.

The new clinical trial will have to investigate which proportion of patients has clinical and possible subclinical disease in the lymph-nodes at the moment of diagnosis, and what role this plays in the prognosis of ovarian carcinoma.

Iatrogenic spread: spill during operation. This is also a subject on which very many conflicting statements have been made. From a theoretical point of view one would assume that a rupture of a tumor with massive spread of tumor cells throughout the peritoneal cavity would result in an increased incidence of peritoneal implants. Although some authors did not find this detrimental effect,[42] there seems to be a general consensus that prognosis is worse after spill, and in these cases a more aggressive treatment is usually recommended.

Webb et al.[101] found that intracapsular processes of stage I (being stage Ia$_1$) carried an excellent prognosis (90% five-year survival). Survival was much lower for extracystic tumors (68%) and adherent (50%) or ruptured (58%) processes. A clear influence of rupture of tumors of stage I during operation would thus only be found for processes which were intracystic. All conditions in which tumor cells are liable to be shed within the peritoneal cavity would worsen the prognosis to about the same extent.

Hematogenic metastases. Most frequently the main problem in the management of ovarian carcinoma is to control the disease in pelvis and abdomen.

In an autopsy series,[10] it appears that in patients in whom the treatment has failed, distant metastases can be found in almost any site but most frequently in lymph nodes, the pleura, the lungs, the liver, and the skeleton.

However, when the disease is locally cured it is very rare to see hematogenic metastases. Rutledge[87] found 26 patients out of a series of 260 who had distant metastases and a local recurrence. Only five patients (about 2%) developed metastases with local control.

Implications of the Biology of Ovarian Tumors for Staging and Treatment

From these data it appears that probably the greatest problem in ovarian carcinoma up to now has been the exact evaluation of the tumor extent.[83] The small transversal incision in the lower abdomen which was very often used for resection and staging of patients with ovarian carcinoma obviously does not allow for a thorough inspection of the upper abdomen, especially the diaphragmatic surface. This was probably done with the idea that peritoneal metastases would move progressively through the abdomen. Absence of peritoneal implants in the lower abdomen was usually accepted as evidence that no macroscopic seeding in the whole peritoneal cavity was present. However, the data from Bagley et al.,[7] and Rosenoff et al.[82] suggest that very often the lower abdomen can be skipped and that diaphragmatic metastases can be the only manifestation of abdominal disease. In 7 patients out of 16 who were originally classified as stage I or II, unsuspected disease was found on the diaphragm immediately after the laparotomy.[82]

The incidence and the role of lymphatic metastases are not clearly defined as yet, but in view of the data available further investigation of this aspect of this disease seems mandatory.

Within the patient group with stages I or II a group should be determined with a high risk of subclinical nodal disease. Extension of the radiotherapy to the para-aortic nodes should be considered in the postoperative treatment of these patients.

The repercussions of these new data on tumor spread will be very important for the prognosis and the treatment of ovarian cancer. The disappointing results obtained until now for disease stage I or II could very well be explained by the fact that some of these patients were hidden stages III. Exact staging will thus result in a redistribution of the patients over the different stages, with even less stages I and II than before and more patients in stage III. This should improve the prognosis of all three of these groups of patients, as stage III should now contain many patients with limited disease.

The underestimation in the past of the tumor extent means that most of the older data on the radiotherapy in the treatment of ovarian carcinoma are only of limited value. Whenever tumor localizations are present outside the treatment field (diaphragm or lymph nodes) this would inevitably lead to failure of the radiotherapy. This is especially true when irradiation was limited to the pelvis, but even with total abdominal irradiation only a relatively low dose is given to the diaphragm, in order to spare the liver.

The better staging procedures will not only help in the choosing of the modality of treatment after surgery but also in deciding the degree of aggressiveness one is willing to use, as the fraction of patients at risk for recurrence directly determines the burden one is willing to place on the whole patient group.

All this means that careful and extensive staging is the absolute prerequisite in any new study on ovarian carcinoma to obtain meaningful information.

Prognostic Factors Other Than Stage of the Disease

Although everyone agrees that the extent of the disease is the single most important prognostic factor, it will be mandatory to take other factors into account in trying to determine some high- and low-risk groups within these stages. The most important ones which have been suggested until now are histological type and degree of differentiation of the tumor, amount of tumor remaining after surgery, and the presence of ascites.

Histologic type. The epithelial tumors are usually subdivided into five groups: the serous, mucinous, endometriod, and mesonephric adenocarcinomas, and the undifferentiated carcinomas. The largest group of these is made up of the serous cystadenocarcinomas, which comprises about 50% of all epithelial malignancies of the ovaries. Cure rate and survival time are significantly lower in serous adenocarcinomas and undifferentiated processes than in the other types,[4,53] but this can be correlated to a large extent with the fact that these processes are much more frequently (75%) diagnosed in late stages (III or IV) than mucinous or endometriod processes, where only 20% of the patients have advanced disease at the moment of diagnosis.[4,59] Although some tumor types thus seem to behave in a more aggressive way, the influence of histologic type independent of stage at diagnosis is not yet clear.

Degree of differentiation. Tumors with a high degree of de-differentiation will have a more aggressive behavior and will more often be diagnosed in late stages.

Several authors[42,54,59,102] find a definite deleterious effect of a lower degree of differentiation even within a certain stage of disease at diagnosis. Other investigators, however, could not confirm this difference.[4,18,70] Malkasian et al.[59] found also that the differences in degree of differentiation were responsible for the influence of the histologic type on prognosis, as the higher malignancy of serous processes was correlated with a lesser degree of differentiation.

Tumor remaining after operation. The possibility of an irradiation or a chemotherapeutic treatment to control malignant disease is correlated to a large extent to the number of cells which have to be killed by either agent. For radiotherapy, it is also known that normal tissue tolerance is determined by the volume of normal tissue encompassed in the radiation fields. The tumor volume which can be controlled by radiotherapy will thus largely be dependent on the tumor spread. This relationship between tumor volume remaining after surgery and prognosis has been described by several authors.[4,22,40,67,92]

From the data from Toronto[23] it would even appear that the extent of the operation is of more importance than the initial stage. When complete resections were done, no difference was found in prognosis for stage I, II, or III after abdomino-pelvic irradiation. This would suggest that the stage would affect the prognosis mainly through its influence on surgical possibilities.

In view of the importance of the residual tumor after surgery it is still widely proposed to do as much debulking as possible even in patients with "inoperable" processes. It seems that prognosis can only be significantly improved if a near-total resection is possible.[67]

Ascites. The meaning of ascites at the time of diagnostic laparotomy has been appraised very differently by several authors. Aure et al. and Parker et al.[73] found that it negatively affected the survival, but this could not be confirmed by Hintz et al.[42] The problem has been rendered even more complex by the latest change in the FIGO classification, where every form of ascites affects the stage of the disease (Ic), while before it was necessary to have malignant cells in the ascites in order to influence the staging. This has probably been done on the assumption that the pathogenesis of ascites is due to tumor infiltration of the diaphragm. A careful examination of the diaphragm could lead to a drastic decrease in the number of patients staged as Ic, bringing a large number of them into stage III and leaving only a small group with subclinical disease in the diaphragm. This is another of the important questions which should be investigated in the near future.

Treatment Modalities

The most important role in the curative treatment of ovarian carcinoma is played by the surgery. Unless a radical or near-total resection can be carried out chances of cure are minimal. However, it has also become apparent that even after such apparently total resections of the tumor, an important fraction of the patients develops a recurrence. Therefore it has been felt necessary to add some form of adjuvant therapy after the surgery. For a long time the only available modality has been radiotherapy, but with the development of the cytostatic drugs many new possibilities are available.

In radiotherapy, one of the basic points is always to define precisely the target area in which the presence of tumor cells is suspected. Also the modalities, such as type of radiation and dose, will be important factors in the effectiveness of the radiotherapy. It appears that a tremendous confusion exists on these points and usually all "irradiated" patients are grouped together without consideration of these factors. The relative importance of these aspects will be discussed.

The search for possible adjuvant therapy with cytostatic drugs is usually done in two stages: first the different drugs are screened on their antitumor effect in patients with advanced disease where regressions can be objectively measured. In a second stage the more effective drugs or combinations thereof are used in an adjuvant situation. The parameter to be evaluated here is no longer tumor growth delay, as it is in patients with advanced disease, but should be the fraction of patients remaining disease-free. These two factors are not always directly linked together, and previous clinical trials involving other tumor sites have revealed that some caution is advisable.

This is the uncertain stage in which the ovarian adjuvant therapy is at this time. As the results of radiotherapy have very often been discouraging in the treatment of a large number of the patients with overt ovarian carcinoma, the advent of chemotherapeutic combinations, which offer definite palliative possibilities, has generated very high hopes that they would be effective in an adjuvant setting, which still has to be proven.

It seems indeed that for patients with advanced disease, which is the majority of the patients, chemotherapy has nearly completely replaced radiotherapy and seems to be more effective. However, this is nearly always palliative treatment and the patient group which requires full attention now is the one with minimal disease after surgery, the very early stages, or those in which only small amounts of tumor had to be left behind.

It is evident that for the moment no clear indications exist for the choice of the treatment modality in these patients. Data are emerging which may explain part of the failures of radiotherapy in the past, while chemotherapy offers possibilities which still have to be confirmed.

More results, especially from prospective clinical studies, will be necessary to determine exactly the role of radiotherapy as well as chemotherapy for these patients.

Surgery. The surgeon has the most important role in the initial management of patients with early stages of ovarian carcinoma. The laparotomy has a double aim: first of all an attempt will be made to remove the tumor from the lower abdomen, and, second, the upper abdomen has to be explored for possible tumor deposits. The importance of this second, diagnostic part of the surgery, for the adjuvant therapy which has to follow has already been stressed. For all cases with stages I and IIa it is usually possible to remove all macroscopic tumor tissue. For a number of the patients with disease in stage IIb this is not possible, as the tumor will have invaded other structures in the pelvis such as the bladder, the bowel, or even the pelvic wall. Residual, macroscopic tumor will, in these cases, be within the well-defined area of the pelvis. Operative techniques have varied in the past from very conservative to radical procedures, but the most common practice now is to perform a bilateral salpingo-oöphorectomy with hysterectomy and omentectomy, although there is no general consensus on the need for this last part.[73,86,103]

For patients in whom a radical procedure is not possible maximal debulking has usually been advised. There is no evidence however that this improves survival significantly unless a nearly total resection is possible.[55,73] Thus an aggressive approach with removal of parts of bowel or colon is only warranted if all tumor masses can be excised.

Radiotherapy. For a long time radiotherapy was the only form of additional treatment after operation. It is impossible to draw any conclusions about the efficacy of radiotherapy in early stages of the disease, as no prospective, randomized series have been carried out, and all series of irradiated patients consist of selected cases with bad prognostic signs. Also, many series still employ orthovoltage irradiation, while it is only since megavoltage apparatus has become available that efficient radiotherapy over large volumes could be given.

In the evaluation of a radiotherapeutic treatment one has always to consider the various parameters involved, such as volume treated, total dose, and type of radiation.

In most of the published series the radiotherapeutic treatment was given with external beams and limited to the pelvis. A few groups, and increasingly so in recent years, have irradiated the total abdominal cavity with external beams. Also, a small number of centers tries to achieve the treatment of the peritoneal cavity by instilling radioactive isotopes, which emit mainly low-energy electrons.

The effectiveness of a certain radiation dose in sterilizing a tumor is directly correlated to the intrinsic radiosensitivity of the tumor cells and to the number of cells in the mass. Larger tumors thus require higher radiation doses.[33] The allowable radiation dose is determined by the radiosensitivity, and also very much by the volume, of normal tissues included in the irradiation fields. The tolerance decreases rapidly for larger treatment volumes. This means that larger tumor masses or multiple localizations influence the therapeutic margin of the radiotherapy by reducing the tolerance as well as by increasing the dose necessary for tumor control. A sound approach in selecting patients for radiotherapy requires a careful evaluation of these different factors.

First, the available data on the role of radiotherapy in postoperative treatment of ovarian carcinoma will be reviewed. On the basis of these data and new ideas on the biology of ovarian cancer, different possible approaches of radiotherapy will be discussed.

No data have been obtained from prospective trials, and the results from retrospective studies are biased due to patient selection. A patient is, in most cases, referred for irradiation by the gynecologist, usually because of known or suspected irradicality of the operation, or because of the bad prognostic signs, such as poor differentiation, rupture of a cyst, or extracystic involvement. For *patients in stage I* a lot of controversy still exists about the use of postoperative radiotherapy, and no beneficial effect has been established as yet. Results are widely divergent in the different series, with five-year survivals of unirradiated patients ranging from 55 to 88%. The irradiated patients do not seem to do any better, with survivals of 40 to 80%.[5,19,21,67,84] The fact that the irradiated patients, who were selected on negative prognostic signs, did as well as the other patients, has been used to demonstrate the efficacy of radiotherapy. This type of argument, however, is too weak to be acceptable. Some of the more recently published series of patients in stage I who were treated with aggressive radiotherapy have fairly good survivals. In the series of Fuks and Bagshaw[36] no extra precautions were taken for accurate staging and all patients were irradiated over the pelvis only. Five-year survival was 85% for Ia and 72% for Ib. Kuipers[57] obtained a three-year survival of 80% for patients in stage I. In the M.D. Anderson Hospital, staging procedures were more strict, and irradiation was given over the pelvis and the whole abdomen. After four years 85% of the patients remain free of disease. From these results it appears that survival of patients with ovarian carcinoma stage I can be raised far above the average of 60%, which was obtained in many series up to a few years ago, but it is not yet clear whether this is primarily due to patient selection after more extensive staging procedures or to more efficient treatment.

A few randomized studies have recently tried to evaluate the influence of adjuvant therapy in patients with stage I. However, most of these studies compare different modalities of adjuvant therapies, and only one has included a group of patients who did not receive any additional therapy. In the trial of the Gynaecologic Oncology Group (GOG)[46,47] no significant differences have been found until now between a melphalan treatment, pelvic irradiation, or no adjuvant therapy. However, follow-up is still short, many patients were excluded from the trial due to protocol violations, and diagnostic procedures to evaluate the upper abdomen were not very strict, so that probably some stage III patients were included.

The best evidence for the efficacy of radiotherapy in the treatment of ovarian carcinoma can be found in the results obtained with *patients with disease in stage II*. This seems to be a group of patients with a high risk of local recurrence within a well-defined target area (pelvis), which can be irradiated with a relatively high dose. Although again no prospective randomized studies are available, all series in which radiotherapy was given show superior results over the patient groups that had only operations.[19,51,67,84]

Distinctions should be made among the stage II patients according to the mass of the remaining tumor after surgery. The main benefit of radiotherapy seems to be obtained in patients where only small numbers of tumor cells have to be sterilized by the radiation. Ovarian cancers are only moderately sensitive to ionizing radiation, and experience has taught that bulky disease can only very seldom be controlled by doses tolerated by the tissues in the pelvis. It has therefore recently become the practice in many centers to try to reduce the tumor mass with chemotherapy before giving the pelvic irradiation. No data are available yet how far this policy is successful.

Prognosis for *patients in stage III* is very poor, and radiotherapy seems to influence the survival fraction very little. However, a small percentage of patients seems to benefit from aggressive radiotherapy,[37] and most of these patients had only a small tumor mass left after surgery. More extensive staging will probably find more of such patients with "very limited" stage III disease who could benefit from radiotherapy.

Very little data are available on the relative value of the *different modalities of radiotherapy*. Most of the series use pelvic irradiations with doses around 5,000 rad. A few extended the radiation fields to the para-aortic nodes[36,37] or the whole abdomen.[14,91] On theoretical grounds the extension of the radiation fields seems very logical, and it is supported by some authors with much experience in this field.[87]

The best evidence in support of the extended radiation fields was obtained by the Toronto group, which compared pelvic irradiation to abdomino-pelvic irradiation or a combination of radiotherapy over the pelvis followed by chemotherapy (Chlorambucil, 6 mg/day, during two years.)[14] Only patients with minimal disease after surgery were included: stage Ib, II, and III, in whom the total planned operative procedure could be carried out (bilateral salpingo-oöphorectomy and hysterectomy, BSOH), and for stage III the additional condition was set that the patients had to be free of any symptoms due to tumor activity six weeks after surgery.

The first analysis[14] showed superior results for all treatment groups receiving treatment outside the pelvis (chemotherapy or irradiation). In stage III, abdominal irradiation was superior to Chorambucil if a "complete BSOH" was done. In another group of stage III patients, where an "incomplete BSOH" was done, prognosis was much worse, and no difference was found between abdominal irradiation and Chlorambucil. This is again an indication that the selection of patients is extremely important and that radiotherapy should probably be reserved for patients with minimal disease.

A very interesting fact emerged from the second analysis of the same patient group, with longer follow-up.[23] The advantage which was initially found through the addition of Chlorambucil to the pelvic irradiation is completely lost, as these patients have their relapses with a delay of about seven to eight months in comparison to those patients only receiving pelvic irradiation. In this study abdomino-pelvic irradiation thus gave the best results. These results will be discussed more extensively in the chapter on chemotherapy.

In a study at the M.D. Anderson Hospital abdomino-pelvic irradiation was compared to Melphalan treatment in patients with stage I, II, and minimal stage III.[99] No significant differences were found for the total group with a five-year survival of 71.5% after irradiation and 78% after Melphalan treatment. Chemotherapy shows a slight advantage in stages I and III, while in stage II radiotherapy results in a superior survival rate.[85] On the basis of these data, these authors favor the chemotherapy as carrying a lesser burden for the patient.

It seems that a lot of the negative experiences with abdominal irradiation stem from the fact the patients were not well selected. If the tumor masses in the abdomen exceed two centimeters, tumor control cannot be expected with the tolerated radiation dose.[21,92] In the areas over liver or kidneys no macroscopic tumor implants should be present at all,[87] as the radiation dose there will have to be even lower than in the rest of the abdomen. Irradiation to the upper abdomen thus seems indicated only in situations where minimal or microscopic disease is present. With such strict indications, total abdominal irradiation could be a very effective tool.[23]

Another approach in the treatment of the whole peritoneal surface, which in recent years has not been used extensively, is the *instillation of radioactive isotopes* in the abdomen. The principle is that the radiation emitted (low-energy electrons) is absorbed in the superficial tissue layers, but does not reach the more radiosensitive organs such as bowel, kidney, liver, and bone marrow. Theoretically the instilled isotopes follow the same pattern of distribution as tumor cells which are shed into the peritoneal cavity, and the radiation dose could thus be optimally distributed. Dosimetric studies of a treatment with Au^{198} (150 mci) suggest that the peritoneal serosa would receive 4,000 rad, the omentum 6,000 rad, and the retroperitoneal nodes 7,000 rad.[66,80] Initially this type of therapy was mainly used as a palliative treatment for patients with advanced disease.[20,49] This indication has now been replaced with the more effective cytostatic drugs which have become available.

Several authors[13,64,77] obtained survivals of over 90% for patients in stage Ia with radio-isotope treatment, sometimes in combination with external irradiation. It is impossible to evaluate what the influence of patient selection has been on these results. Aure et al.[5] reported from a retrospective study that the addition of radioactive gold to an external irradiation improved the survival from 63 to 84%. In a nonrandomized study Decker et al.[20] found a beneficial effect of radiogold treatment in patients where a rupture had occurred during the operation (five-year survival was 80% vs. 43% for a matched group). In a prospective randomized trial[53] an advantage in the addition of radioactive gold was found in patients with stage I, where tumor rupture had occurred during operation, and a slight benefit in stage II. Unfortunately, a large part of these better results on the tumor were lost by the high incidence in intercurrent deaths due to treatment complications, which has led the Norwegian group to drop the external radiation in patients receiving the intraperitoneal isotopes.

Such severe and even fatal complications are found in several series, especially when the isotope instillation was associated with external irradiation.[20,44,81,99] After this type of treatment there is usually extensive fibrosis of the serosa with multiple adhesions. Complications are most frequently obstruction and fistula formation, and surgical interventions are very difficult.

Although it thus seems that intra-abdominal isotope instillations could be of some benefit, the indications should be limited to patients who do not require external radiation (after radical operations), in centers which have some experience with such type of treatments. Randomized clinical trials are necessary to determine its indications and real potential.

Some authors[36,57] have proposed that extension of the radiation field beyond the pelvis might in some cases be limited to the para-aortic nodes instead of including the whole abdomen. This would have the advantage of allowing the use of higher radiation doses, as the volume of normal tissue included is much smaller. Evidently this policy would only be of benefit in patient groups in which there is a sizeable fraction with subclinical nodal disease and where there is very little risk of a tumor recurrence in the upper abdomen. It seems at the present time that no patient group can be selected that would be at risk for the lymph nodes but not for the peritoneal cavity. The upper abdomen would thus have to be treated either with irradiation or with chemotherapy. It would seem that a booster radiation dose to the lumbo-aortic nodes over a total abdominal irradiation would not be tolerated, so that this type of irradiation would probably always have to be combined with some chemotherapeutic treatment.

Although such combination treatments may offer definite possibilities, it seems that it is more urgent to answer the basic questions on the efficacy of radiotherapy or chemotherapy in the curative treatment of ovarian carcinoma before trying to evaluate more complex questions in clinical trials.

The situation is somewhat different in patients who have demonstrated invasion of the lymph nodes. In some of these patients the nodal involvement is the only tumor localization otuside the pelvis, and if this is small (e.g., with only positive nodal biopsies), it seems that radiotherapy of regional lymph nodes must be included in their treatment. If, however, the nodes are bulky, experience in cervical carcinoma would suggest that prognosis is dismal and even chances for local control are low.

In view of the evidence of early invasion of the diaphragm, inclusion of this organ in the irradiated volume has also been proposed.[38] The same arguments are valid here as already given for nodal irradiation. It seems attractive in situations where the diaphragm is the only known site of tumor, but its role in an adjuvant setting remains to be tested, and this should probably be done only in conjunction with chemotherapy.

Chemotherapy. Nearly all available data concern the effectiveness of different drugs or combinations thereof on advanced disease. The efficacy is usually measured by means of regression of clinically evauable tumor masses and by the duration of a remission. Hardly any data are available on the role of these drugs in an adjuvant setting.

The most extensively investigated drugs for the treatment of ovarian carcinoma are the alkylating agents.[109] In different series, initial objective regression rates have varied from 35 to 65%, with 5 to 15% of all initially treated patients still responding to treatment two years after the beginning of the therapy. No significant difference could be demonstrated among the different drugs used, the mode of administration (orally or intravenously), or the dose distribution (continuous or pulse).[108] The intraperitoneal administration of the drug does not seem to be superior and may even be less effective than the intravenous method.[39,93]

Treatment results are definitely better in patients who did not receive other treatment beforehand. There is no influence of the histology on the fraction of tumors going into re-gression,[9,39] but in the undifferentiated processes there are less complete regressions and the length of the remissions are shorter.[93] In patients with a good initial response to che-motherapy, survival is definitely higher than in patients who do not react well to the drugs.[60,93] In these patients with advanced disease, chemotherapy is continued until clinical relapse. The necessity of this policy was demonstrated by the fact that in patients who were clinically in complete remission, very often tumor was found at second-look surgery[93] or, when treatment was discontinued, a very rapid relapse occurred.[9,61] This stresses the fact that in an elective setting the results of chemotherapy can only be evaluated with sufficient follow-up after discontinuing the treatment.

The possibilities of nonalkylating agents have been much less investigated in the past, and it is only very recently that some progress has been made. Very often they have been tested in patients who did not respond to alkylating agents, which makes it difficult to in-terpret the results. Most experience has been gathered with 5-FU, which achieves regression rates in about 30% of the patients.[2,58,98]

Adriamycin seems to give results comparable to those obtained with alkylating agents,[8,72] and there seems to be no cross resistance with this type of drug, which would offer interesting prospects for combined treatments.

Another promising drug for this disease seems to be hexamethylmelamine, which also has no cross resistance with alkylating agents.[100,104] In a recent study in the M.D. Anderson Hospital hexamethylmelamine produced superior results to Melphalan.[90]

A last interesting drug is CDDP (cisdiamine dichloride platinum), which is rather toxic,[105,106] but has shown interesting possibilities.

The early attempts at treatment with combination chemotherapy were only moderately successful. No difference in survival was found between two groups of patients treated either with Melphalan only or with a combination of cyclophosphamide, 5-fluorouracil and ac-tinomycin D. Toxicity, however, was much higher with the combination treatment.[92,94] A combination of 5-FU, Methotrexate and Cytoxan also did no better than Melphalan alone (trial of the ECOG, Eastern Cooperative Oncology Group). Cytoxan alone had the same results as in combination with adriamycin in one study,[27] but encouraging results (46% complete remissions) were obtained recently with this combination.[75,97] However, no ad-vantage in survival level was obtained.

Recently, combinations of hexamethylmelamine with Cytoxan seemed to give very good results in M.D. Anderson Hospital.[62] This drug has also been given in combination with 5-FU, methotrexate and cyclophosphamide (Hexa-CAF).[107] Also, CDDP (cis-platinum) has shown interesting possibilities in combination with adriamycin[12] or with adriamycin and Cytoxan.[28]

Altogether, it seems that drug combinations that are more toxic than single agents have not been demonstrated to be significantly more effective in treating advanced stages of ovarian carcinoma.[62] A great effort is being made in this field now, and encouraging results have been obtained recently, but due to very short follow-up it is still impossible to judge what the impact of the new chemotherapy schemes will be on adjuvant treatment.

Although very little attention has been paid to hormonal treatment of ovarian cancer, some studies describe a low frequency (10%) of remission induction, but surprisingly, some of them have been longlasting. In some ovarian tumors progesterone receptors have been demonstrated, so that a selection could be made of patients who could benefit from this type of treatment.

All the results described above have been obtained in patients with advanced disease. Such studies are necessary in order to select some drugs or combinations of drugs that have definite effect on a certain type of tumor. These drugs or combinations can then be used in an adjuvant setting in patients who very often have no clinically evaluable disease.

The data on the value of chemotherapy as an adjuvant treatment in early stages of ovarian carcinoma are even more scarce than those on radiotherapy and as difficult to interpret. In comparison to radiotherapy, there is an additional problem in evaluating adjuvant chemotherapy in the length of the treatment. Irradiation is given immediately after surgery and is finished in a few weeks. All remaining tumor cells will begin to proliferate at the end of the treatment and, if the patient is not tumor-free, a recurrence will soon become clinically detectable. This is not so for chemotherapy, as this is usually given for one or two years and sometimes even longer. Even if the drug succeeds only partially, tumor can remain below the level of clinical detection during the maintenance therapy and may only be detected after discontinuation of therapy. Two different parameters should thus always be considered: first, the time during which the patient can be kept symptom-free or alive, including the time of treatment, and second and most important, the fraction of patients who remain disease-free when treatment is stopped.

The first parameter, symptom-free interval or length of survival, is mainly palliative and a balance between the burden on the patient and the gain in survival time must always be considered. In adjuvant treatment, where one is not looking for gain in survival time but in survival fraction, not many data are available. In a nonrandomized study, Julian and Woodruff[48] gave 14 patients with stage I disease a five-week treatment of Chlorambucil after surgery. Thirteen of these patients remained disease-free. Nye[69] found no improvement in survival by treating localized disease with triethylene thiophosphoramide when comparing 175 patients with matched historical controls. The GOG study[47] compares Melphalan or pelvic irradiation to no adjuvant treatment and has not yet demonstrated a significant difference. The study in Toronto suggested, at first analysis,[14] a definite advantage in adding Chlorambucil to pelvic irradiation in patients with stage I or II disease. After longer follow-up however, survival in the two groups is similar and an advantage in the chemotherapy is no longer found.

In the M.D. Anderson equal survivals are found for patients treated with Melphalan or abdomino-pelvic irradiation for the total group of patients with stage I, II, or minimal stage III.[91] When evaluated separately, chemotherapy did better in stages I and III and radiotherapy in stage II.

Practical Guidelines for Management of Early Stages of Ovarian Carcinoma

As too many factors remain uncertain, it is not possible to stipulate a single good policy for the treatment of the different stages of ovarian carcinoma. An attempt will be made to discuss the different possible therapeutic attitudes, their rationale, and their possibilities.

One can consider as "early stages" all patients in whom the tumor can be radically or nearly totally resected. This would include all stages I, many stages II, and a few stages III. The decision whether to give adjuvant therapy or not, the choice of the modality, and the aggressiveness of the treatment is largely dependent on the natural prognosis of the disease. As has already been said, staging procedures have changed quite a bit lately, and this means that some uncertainty now exists about this prognosis for the different stages, and especially the early ones, making decisions for adjuvant therapy even more difficult.

Stage Ia$_1$. The general consensus seems to be that for processes limited to one ovary, which grow intracapsularly and which have not ruptured during operation, prognosis seems to be excellent and no adjuvant therapy is necessary.

Stages Ia$_2$, Ib, and IIa. Prognosis for these three groups seems very similar. All conditions in which a unilateral tumor has an increased chance to shed cells into the peritoneal cavity definitely influence prognosis. Bilateral tumors or invasion of the genitalia interna also detract from the prognosis. Results would seem to vary between 60 and 80%, which definitely would require adjuvant therapy. No data exist to confirm the value of either radiotherapy or chemotherapy in these stages. No good evidence exists as to whether most of these patients fail in the pelvis or in the abdomen. In the Toronto study, treatment outside the pelvis influenced the time of the recurrence (Chlorambucil) and even the incidence of failing patients (abdominal irradiation). However, stages IIb were also included in this group. These are the patients for which the greatest uncertainty exists for therapy selection.

Radiotherapeutic modalities could be irradiation of the pelvis to a high dose, irradiation of the whole peritoneal cavity to a somewhat lower dose, or a combination of both (abdominal irradiation with boost to the pelvis). Irradiation of the whole abdomen can be given by external irradiation, by *strip irradiation* by *open-field technique,* or by instillation of radioactive isotopes.

Strip irradiation is much more difficult and does not seem to give better results than open-field technique.[30,36,76] Isotope instillation could have interesting possibilities, but it is also a difficult technique, carrying a fair risk of complications, and should probably be left to a few experienced centers to be further tested.

The choice would then be between limited or extended open-field irradiation. The very good results of Toronto and Houston with whole-abdomen irradiation and the disappointing results with pelvic irradiation would suggest the extended field as more appropriate. The Canadian group does offer some good evidence that extension of the radiation field outside the pelvis improves the results. However, both these studies are fairly recent, and the improved survivals were probably also due to more accurate staging.

In evaluating the results of abdomino-pelvic irradiation, it appears that many complications come from the booster dose to the pelvis. As there is no evidence that in these stages the pelvis is more at risk than the rest of the abdomen, one could imagine that the whole abdomen and pelvis could be irradiated to the same dose without boost to the pelvis. However, this has never been done before and should only be tested in a randomized study.

This concept is comparable to that of the prophylactic lung irradiation in osteosarcoma, which was tested in a randomized trial by the radiotherapy/chemotherapy group of the EORTC.[11] It is based on the fact that radiotherapy, when given in low doses, has a certain chance of sterilizing microscopic deposits of tumor, as they are more radiosensitive and contain only very small numbers of cells. The radiation tolerance of the abdomen being greater than that of the lung, and ovarian carcinoma being somewhat more radiosensitive than osteosarcoma, the same policy could also be successful.

The uncertainties about the role of chemotherapy in these stages of the disease are the same as for radiotherapy. No hard evidence is available to show that the surviving fraction is ultimately higher when patients receive adjuvant chemotherapy. Here also the good results obtained could be due to better staging procedures. The available results would suggest that in this group of patients alkylating agents are still the best choice for adjuvant therapy, as they produce high percentages of remissions with moderate toxicity in patients with advanced disease.

The possible greater effectiveness of polychemotherapeutic regimes has not yet been solidly enough confirmed to balance their much higher toxicity in this patient group with a reasonable prognosis.

In the choice between radiotherapy and chemotherapy, the side effects of the two treatment modalities have to be taken into account. It was usually accepted that radiotherapy carried a larger burden for the patients than alkylating agents. However, evaluation after longer follow-up of patients having received Melphalan or Chlorambucil revealed a definitely increased incidence of leukemia.[23,29] As the numbers are fairly small, some caution is necessary in the interpretation of these data, but they should be kept in mind when treating patients with a high chance of long-term survival.

Stages Ic, IIb and III. Here more evidence seems available. These patients (certainly all stages IIb and stages III, which showed invasion of the pelvic structures) have a very high chance of pelvic recurrence. Data from the literature support pelvic irradiation as an effective tool in treating this stage of the disease, probably due to a decrease in the number of local recurrences.

However, it also seems that extension of the treatment to the upper abdomen is necessary. While Smith et al.[90] found that chemotherapy is as effective as radiotherapy, Dembo et al.[23,24] showed that irradiation was more effective than treatment with a single alkylating agent (Chlorambucil).

In view of the much worse prognosis of these patients, there is a tendency to combine radiotherapy and chemotherapy. It still seems justified, however, to make a choice between irradiation of the upper abdomen or chemotherapy as an adjunct to the pelvic irradiation. The lesser prognosis could justify the use of a more toxic combination treatment of chemotherapy. This is especially so in cases where not only subclinical disease is to be eradicated, but where macroscopic tumor nodules have been left behind at surgery. In view of the problems of controlling bulky disease in the pelvis with radiotherapy, some centers now try to reduce the mass before irradiation with combination chemotherapy.

CONCLUSION

Based on the available data it is impossible to set strict guidelines for the treatment of patients with early stages of ovarian carcinoma. Due to the disappointing experience in the past with radiotherapy and the demonstration of the effectiveness of some chemo-therapeutic regimens in palliative treatment, there has been a profound change in the policy used in many centers. Some authors have even suggested that chemotherapy could totally replace radiotherapy, which would have no more place in the management of this disease.

Although it seems that this is largely so in palliative treatment where radiotherapy can only rarely hope to achieve good clinical remissions in patients with diffuse and bulky disease, this should by no means be extrapolated to the curative treatment in early stages. There is strong evidence that radiotherapy is effective in suppressing pelvic recurrences in patients who show signs of local invasion (stage II or III). There is preliminary evidence that radiotherapy could be very effective in controlling disease in the upper abdomen if only patients with minimal disease are treated.

In two studies, alkylating agents were suggested to do as well as radiotherapy. However, on longer follow-up one of these studies showed an advantage for radiotherapy. This stresses again the fact that follow-up periods should be long enough after discontinuation of therapy before drawing conclusions.

The further evaluation of the effectiveness of radiotherapy will require careful selection of the target volume. This could be the pelvis, the lumbo-aortic nodes, the diaphragm, or the whole peritoneal cavity. It should be borne in mind that the tolerance is related to the volume irradiated, and it is thus always necessary to choose between large volume/low dose or small volume/high dose irradiations.

Chemotherapy has shown its ability to induce tumor regressions and to delay recurrences. Its ability to increase the fraction of cured patients is still to be confirmed, but initial results look encouraging. In treatment with drugs, there is no problem in selecting target volumes as in radiotherapy. The main point of investigation here is the evaluation of the effectiveness of new drugs or combinations.

Although the main question in patients with subclinical disease after surgery is still the indication for radiotherapy or chemotherapy, it seems that in those patients with larger amounts of residual disease (diameter more than 2–3 cm) both these agents will be necessary. Neither radiotherapy nor chemotherapy when used alone seems to have a good chance of controlling such tumors. For these patients the question will be how best to combine both these agents to obtain the greatest effectiveness.

Progress will only be obtained when these different questions are approached in a systematic way and with an open mind by the people involved in these different fields.

REFERENCES

1. American Cancer Society (1975). *Cancer Facts and Figures,* New York.
2. Ansfield, F.J.; Shroeder, J.M.; and Curreri A.R. (1962). Five years clinical experience with 5-Fluorouracil. *J Am Med Assoc,* 181:295–99.
3. Athey, P.A.; Wallace S.; Jing, B-S.; Gallager, H.S.; and Smith J.P. (1975). Lymphangiography in ovarian cancer. *Am J Roentgenol,* 123:106–113.
4. Aure, J.A.; Hoeg, K.; and Kolstad P. (1971a). Clinical and histologic studies of ovarian carcinoma: long term follow-up of 990 cases. *Obstet Gynecol,* 37:1–9.

5. Aure, J.C.; Hoeg, K.; and Kolstad, P. (1971b). Radioactive colloidal gold in the treatment of ovarian carcinoma. *Acta Radiol (Ther)*, **10**:399–407.

6. Bagley, C.M., Young, R.C.; Canellos, G.P.; and De Vita, V.T. (1972). Treatment of ovarian carcinoma: possibilities for progress. *N Engl J Med*, **287**:856–62.

7. Bagley, C.M.; Young, R.C.; Schein, P.S.; Chabner, B.A.: and De Vita, V.T. (1973). Ovarian carcinoma metastatic to the diaphragm—frequently undiagnosed at laparotomy. *Am J Obstet Gynecol*, **116**:397–400.

8. Barlow, J.J.; Piver, M.S.; Chuang, J.T.; Cortes, E.P.; Ohnuma, T.; and Holland, J.F. (1973). Adriamycin and bleomycin alone and in combination in gynecologic cancers. *Cancer*, **32**:735–41.

9. Beck, R.E.; and Boyes, D.A. (1968). Treatment of 126 cases of advanced ovarian carcinoma with cyclophosphamide. *Cancer Med Assoc J*, **98**:539–41.

10. Bergman, F. (1966). Carcinoma of the ovary. *Acta Obstet Gynecol Scand*, **45**:211–31.

11. Breur, K.; Cohen, P.; Schweisguth, O.; and Hart, A.M.M. (1978). Irradiation of the lungs as an adjuvant therapy in the treatment of osteosarcoma of the limbs: an EORTC randomized study. *Europ J Cancer*, **14**:461–71.

12. Bruckner, H.W.; Cohen, C.J.; Gusberg, S.B.; Wallach, R.C.; Kabakow, B.; Greenspan, E.M.; and Holland J.F. (1976). Chemotherapy of ovarian cancer with adriamycin (ADM) and cis-platinum (DDP). *Proc Am Soc Clin Oncol*, **17**:287.

13. Buchsbaum, H.J.; Keettel, W.C.; and Latourette, H.B. (1975). The use of radioisotopes as adjunct therapy of localized ovarian cancer. *Seminars in Oncology*, **2**:247–51.

14. Bush, R.S.; Allt, W.E.C.; Beale, F.A.; Bean, H.; Springle, J.F.; and Sturgeon, J. (1977). Treatment of epithelial carcinoma of the ovary: operation, irradiation, and chemotherapy. *Am J Obstet Gynecol*, **127**:692–704.

15. Coates, G.; Bush, R.S.; and Aspin, N. (1973). A study of ascites using lymphoscintigraphy with ^{99m}Tc-sulphur colloid. *Radiol*, **107**:577–83.

16. Courtice, F.C.; and Steinbeck, A.W. (1950). The lymphatic drainage of plasma from the peritoneal cavity of the cat. *Austr J Exp Biol Med Sci*, **28**:161–82.

17. Cutler, S.J.; Myers, M.H.; and Green, S.B. (1975). Trends in survival rates of patients with cancer. *N Engl J Med*, **293**:122–124.

18. Czernobilski, B.; Silverman, B.B.; and Mikuta, J.J. (1970). Endometrioid carcinoma of the ovary: a clinicopathologic study of 75 cases. *Cancer* **26**:1141–52.

19. Dalley, V.M. (1969). Radiotherapy in malignant disease of the ovary. *Proc R Soc Med* **62**:359–361.

20. Decker, D.G.; Webb, M.J.; and Holbrook, M.A. (1973). Radiogold treatment of epithelial cancer of ovary: late results. *Am J Obstet Gynecol*, **115**:751–56.

21. Delclos, L., and Smith, J.P. (1973). Tumors of the ovary. In *Textbook of Radiotherapy*, Fletcher G., (Ed.), Lea and Febiger, Philadelphia.

22. Delclos, L., and Quinlan, E. (1969). Malignant tumors of the ovary managed with postoperative megavoltage irradiation. *Radiol*, **93**:659–63.

23. Dembo, A.J.; Bush, R.S.; Beale, F.A.; Bean, H.A.; Pringle, J.F.; and Sturgeon, J. (1978). Improved survival with abdomino-pelvic irradiation in patients with carcinoma of the ovary, stages Ib, II, asymptomatic III, BSOH-completed. *Am Soc Clin Oncol*, Abstr. C-74.

24. Dembo, A.J.; Bush, R.S.: Beale, F.A.; Bean, H.A.; Pringle, J.F.; Sturgeon, J.; and Reid, J.G. (in press). Ovarian carcinoma: improved survival following abdomino-pelvic irradiation in patients with a completed pelvic operation. *Am J Obstet Gynecol*.

25. Douglas, B.; McDonald, J.S.; and Baker, J.W. (1971). Lymphography in carcinoma of the ovary. *Proc R Soc Med* **64**:400–401.

26. Drye, J.C. (1948). Intraperitoneal pressure in the human. *Surg Gynecol Obstet* **87**:472–475.

27. Edmonson, J.H. (1975). Status report of Mayo Clinic studies. *Natl Cancer Inst Monogr* **42**:167–168.

28. Ehrlich, C.E.; Einhorn, L.H.; and Morgan, J.L. (1978). Combination chemotherapy of ovarian carcinoma with Cis-diamminedichloroplatinum (CDDP), Adriamycin (ADR) and Cytoxan (CTX). *Proc Am Soc Clin Oncol* **292**.

29. Einhorn, N. (1978). Acute leukemia after chemotherapy (Melphalan). *Cancer* **41**:444–447.

30. Fazekas, J.T.; and Maier, J.G. (1974). Irradiation of ovarian carcinomas. A prospective comparison of the open-field and moving-strip techniques. *Am J Roentgenol* **120**:118–123.

31. Feldman, G.B.; and Knapp, R.C. (1974). Lymphatic drainage of the peritoneal cavity and its significance in ovarian cancer. *Am J Obstet Gynecol* 119:991–994.

32. Feldman, G.B.; Knapp, R.C.; Orden, S.E.; and Hellman, S. (1972). The role of lymphatic obstruction in the formation of ascites in a murine ovarian carcinoma. *Cancer Research* 32:1663–1666.

33. Fletcher, G. (1974). Clinical dose-response curve of subclinical aggregates of epithelial cells and its practical application in the management of human cancer. In *The Biological and Clinical Basis of Radiosensitivity*, Friedman. (Ed.) Thomas, Springfield, pp. 485–501.

34. French, J.E.; Florey, H.W.; and Morris, B.L. (1960). The absorption of particles by the lymphatics of the diaphragm. *Quart J Exp Biol* 45:88–103.

35. Fuchs, W.A. (1969). Malignant tumors of the ovary. In *Recent Results in Cancer Research—Lymphography in Cancer*. Fuchs, W.A.; Davidson, J.W.; and Fisher, H.W. (Eds.). Springer, New York, pp. 119–123.

36. Fuks, Z.; and Bagshaw, M.A. (1975). The rationale for radiotherapy with curative intent for ovarian carcinoma. *Int J Rad Oncol Biol Phys* 1:21–32.

37. Fuks, Z. (1975). External radiotherapy of ovarian cancer: standard approaches and new frontiers. *Semin Oncol* 2:253–266.

38. Glatstein, E.; Fuks, Z.; and Bagshaw; M.A. (1977). Diaphragmatic treatment in ovarian carcinoma: a new radiotherapeutic technique. *Int J Rad Oncol Biol Phys* 2:357–362.

39. Green, T.H. (1959). Hemisulfur mustard in the palliation of patients with metastatic ovarian cancer. *Obstet Gynecol* 13:383–393.

40. Griffiths, C.T.; Grogan, R.H.; and Hall, T.C. (1972). Advanced ovarian cancer: primary treatment with surgery, radiotherapy and chemotherapy. *Cancer* 29:1–7.

41. Hanks, G.E.; and Bagshaw, M.A. (1969). Megavoltage radiation therapy and lymphangiography in ovarian cancer. *Radiol* 93:649–654.

42. Hintz, B.L.; Fuks, Z.; Kempson, R.L.; Eltringham, J.R.; Zaloudek, C.; Williamson, T.J.; and Bagshaw, M.A. (1975). Results of postoperative megavoltage radiotherapy of malignant surface epithelial tumors of the ovary. *Radiol* 114:695–700.

43. Hirabayashi, K.; and Graham, J. (1970). The genesis of ascites in ovarian cancer. *Am J Obstet Gynecol* 106:492–497.

44. Holbrook, M.A.; Welch, J.S.; and Childs, D.S. (1964). Adjuvant use of radioactive colloid in the treatment of carcinoma of the ovary. *Radiol* 83:888–891.

45. Holm-Nielsen, P. (1953). Pathogenesis of ascites in peritoneal carcinomatosis. *Acta Path Microbiol Scand* 33:10–21.

46. Hreshchyshyn, M.M. (1975). Results of the Gynecologic Oncology Group trial on ovarian cancer: preliminary report. *Natl Cancer Inst Monogr* 42:155–165.

47. Hreshchyshyn, M.M.; and Norris, H.J. (1977). Postoperative treatment of women with resectable ovarian cancer with radiotherapy, Melphalan or no further treatment. *Proc Am Assoc Cancer Res* 777, 1977.

48. Julian, C.G; and Woodruff, J.D. (1969). The role of chemotherapy in the treatment of primary ovarian malignancy. *Obstet Gynecol Surv* 24:1307–1342.

49. Keettel, W.C.; and Elkins, H.B. (1956). Experience with radioactive colloidal gold in the treatment of ovarian carcinoma. *Am J Obstet Gynecol* 71:553–568.

50. Keettel, W.C.; and Pixley, E. (1958). Diagnostic value of peritoneal washings. *Clin Obstet Gynecol* 1: 592–606.

51. Kent, S.W.; and McKay, D. G. (1960). Primary cancer of the ovary. *Am J Obstet Gynecol* 80:430–438.

52. Kanpp, R.C.; and Friedman, E.A. (1974). Aortic lymph node metastases in early ovarian cancer. *Am J Obstet Gynecol* 119:1013–1017.

53. Kolstad, P.; Davy, M.; and Hoeg, K. (1977). Individualized treatment of ovarian cancer. *Am J Obstet Gynecol* 128:617–623.

54. Kottmeier, H.L. (1968). Clinical staging in ovarian carcinoma. In: *Ovarian Cancer*, Gentil, F.; and Junqueira, A.C. (Eds.). Springer-Verlag, New York, pp. 146–156.

55. Kottmeier, H.L. (1968). Treatment of ovarian cancer with Thiotepa. *Clin Obstet Gynecol* 11:428–438.

56. Kottmeier, H.L. (Ed.) (1973). Annual report on the results of treatment in carcinoma of the uterus, vagina and ovary. *Int Fed Gynecol Obstet* 15.

57. Kuipers, TJ. (1976). Report on treatment of cancer of the ovary. *Br J Radiol* 49:526–532.

58. Malkasian, G.D.; Decker, D.G.; Mussey, E.; and Johnson, C.E. (1968). Observations on gynecologic malignancy treated with 5-Fluorouracil. *Am J Obstet Gynecol* 100:1012–1017.

59. Malkasian, G.D.; Decker, D.G.; and Webb, M.J. (1975). Histology of epithelial tumors of the ovary: clincal usefulness and prognostic significance of the histologic classification and grading. *Semin Oncol* **2**:191–201.

60. Masterson, J.G. (1967). Management of ovarian carcinoma: surgery, irradiation and chemotherapy. *Am J Obstet Gynecol* **98**:374–386.

61. Masterson, J.G.; and Nelson, J.H. (1965). The role of chemotherapy in the treatment of gynecologic malignancy. *Am J Obstet Gynecol* **93**:1102–1111.

62. McGuire, W.P.; and Young, R.C. (1978). Ovarian cancer. In *Randomized Trial in Cancer: a Critical Review by Sites*. Staquet, M.J. (Ed.). Raven Press, New York, pp. 273–288.

63. Meyers, M.A. (1970). The spread and localization of acute intraperitoneal effusions. *Radiol* **95**:547–554.

64. Moore, D.W.; and Langley, I.I. (1967). Routine use of radiogold following operation for ovarian cancer. *Am J Obstet Gynecol* **98**:624–630.

65. Morton, D.G.; Moore, J.G.; and Chang, N. (1961). The clinical value of peritoneal lavage for cytologic examination. *Am J Obstet Gynecol* **81**:1115–1125.

66. Müller, J.H. (1963). Curative aim and results of routine intraperitoneal radiocolloid administration in the treatment of ovarian carcinoma. *Am J Roentgenol Rad Ther Nucl Med* **89**:533–540.

67. Munnell, W. (1968). The changing prognosis and treatment in cancer of the ovary. *Am J Obstet Gynecol* **100**:790–805.

68. Musumeci, R.; Banfi, A.; Bolis, G.; Battista Candiani, G.; de Palo, G.; DiRe, F.; Luciani, L.; Lattuada, A.; Mangioni, C.; Mattiolo, G.; and Natale, N. (1977). Lymphangiography in patients with ovarian epithelial cancer—an evaluation of 289 consecutive cases. *Cancer* **40**:1444–1449.

69. Nye, E.B. (1972). Ovarian carcinoma: improvement in survival time after chemotherapy. *J Obstet Gynecol Br Commonw* **79**:550–554.

70. Van Orden, D.E.; McAllister, W.B.; Zerne, S.R.M.; and McLean, M.J. (1966). Ovarian carcinoma. The problems of staging and grading. *Am J Obstet Gynecol* **94**:195–202.

71. Overholt, R.H. (1931). Intraperitoneal pressure. *Arch Surg* **22**:691–703.

72. De Palo, G.M.; de Lena, M; DiRe, F.; Luciani, L.; Volagussa, P.; and Bonadonna, G. (1975). Melphalan versus Adriamycin in the treatment of advanced carcinoma of the ovary. *Surg Gynecol Obstet* **141**:899–902.

73. Parker, R.T.; Parker, C.H.; and Wilbanks, G.D. (1970). Cancer of the ovary: survival studies based upon operative therapy, chemotherapy and radiotherapy. *Am J Obstet Gynecol* **108**:878–888.

74. Parker, B.R.; Castellino, R.A.; Fuks, Z.Y.; and Bagshaw, M.A. (1974). The role of lymphography in patients with ovarian cancer. *Cancer* **34**:100–105.

75. Parker, L.M.; Griffiths, C.T.; Yankee, A.; Knapp, R.C.; Canellos, G.P.; and Lokich, J.J. (1978). Adriamycin (A)/Cyclophosphamide (C) and surgical treatment of advanced ovarian cancer. *Proc Am Soc Clin Oncol* **372**.

76. Perez, C.A.; Korba, A.; Zivnuska, F.; Prasad, S.; and Katzenstein, A-L. (1978). [60]Co moving strip technique in the management of carcinoma of the ovary: analysis of tumour control and morbidity. *Int J Rad Oncol Biol Phys* **4**:379–388.

77. Piver, M.S. (1967). Radioactive colloids in the treatment of stage Ia ovarian cancer. *Am J Obstet Gynecol* **98**:624–630.

78. Piver, M.S. (1972). Radioactive colloids in the treatment of stage Ia ovarian cancer. *Obstet Gynecol* **40**:42–44.

79. Raybuck, H.E.; Allen, L.; and Harms, W.S. (1960). Absorption of serum from the peritoneal cavity. *Am J Physiol* **199**:1021–1024.

80. Reed, G.W.; Watson, E.R.; and Chester, M.S. (1961). A note on the distribution of radioactive colloidal gold following intraperitoneal injection. *Br J Radiol* **34**:323–326.

81. Rose, R.G. (1961). Intracavitary radioactive gold in management of ovarian carcinoma. *Obstet Gynecol* **18**:557–563.

82. Rosenoff, S.H.; DeVita, V.T.; Hubbard, S.; and Young, R.C. (1975). Peritoneoscopy in the staging and follow-up of ovarian cancer. *Semin Oncol* **2**:223–228.

83. Rubin, P. (1975). Understanding the problem of understaging in ovarian cancer. *Semin Oncol* **2**:235–242.

84. Rubin, P., Grise, J.W.; and Terry, R. (1962). Has postoperative irradiation proved itself? *Am J Roentgenol* **88:**849–866.

85. Rutledge, F. (1978). Personal communication.

86. Rutledge, F.N.; Fletcher, G.H.; Smith, J.P.; Wharton, J.T.; Delclos, L.; Day, T.G.; and Gallager, N.S. (1976). Gynecologic cancer. In: *Cancer Patient Care at M.D. Anderson Hospital and Tumour Institute, University of Texas*. Clark, R.L. and Howe, C.D. (Eds.). Yearbook Medical Publishers, Chicago, pp. 263–308.

87. Rutledge, F. (1976). Treatment of epithelial cancer of the ovary (Müllerian origin). In: *Gynecologic Oncology*, Rutledge F., Bornow, R.C., and Wharton, J.T. (Eds.). Wiley, New York, pp. 183–199.

88. Scully, R.E. (1970). Recent progress in ovarian cancer. *Human Pathol* **1.**

89. Simer, P.H. (1944). The drainage of particular matter from the peritoneal cavity by lymphatics. *Anat Rec* **88:**175–192.

90. Smith, J.P.; and Rutledge, F.N. (1975). Random study of Hexamethylmelamine, 5-Fluorouracil and Melphalan in treatment of advanced carcinoma of the ovary. *Natl Cancer Inst Monogr* **42:**169–172.

91. Smith, J.P.; Rutledge, F.N.; and Delclos, L. (1975). Results of chemotherapy as an adjunct to surgery in patients with localized ovarian cancer. *Semin Oncol* **2:**277–281.

92. Smith, J.P.; Rutledge, F.N.; and Wharton, J.T. (1972). Chemotherapy of ovarian cancer: new approaches to treatment. *Cancer* **30:**1565–1571.

93. Smith, J.P.; and Rutledge, F.N. (1970). Chemotherapy in the treatment of cancer of the ovary. *Am J Obstet Gynecol* **107:**691–703.

94. Smith, J.P.; and Rutledge, F.N. (1973). Metastatic ovarian cancer. *Clin Obstet Gynecol* **16:**286–297.

95. Tobias, J.S.; and Griffiths; C.T. (1976). Management of ovarian carcinoma. *N Engl J Med* **294:**818–823.

96. Tobias, J.S.; and Griffiths, C.T. (1976). Management of ovarian carcinoma. *N Engl J Med* **294:**877–882.

97. Turbow, M.M.; Fuks, Z.; and Glatstein, E. (1978). Chemotherapy of ovarian carcinoma: randomization between Melphalan and Adriamycin-Cyclophosphamide. *Proc Am Soc Clin Oncol* **349.**

98. Vaitevicius, V.K.; Brennan, M.J.; Beckett, V.L.; Kelly, J.E.; and Talley, R.W. (1961). Clinical evaluation of cancer chemotherapy with 5-Fluorouracil. *Cancer* **14:**131–135.

99. Villasanta, U.; and Bloedorn, F.G. (1968). Operation, external irradiation, radioactive isotopes and chemotherapy in the treatment of metastatic ovarian malignancies. *Am J Obstet Gynecol* **102:**531–536.

100. Wampler, G.L.; Mellette, S.J.; Kuperminc, M.; and Regelson, W. (1972). Hexamethylmelamine (NSC—13785) in the treatment of advanced cancer. *Cancer Chemother Rep* **56:**505–514.

101. Webb, M.J.; Decker, D.G.; Mussey, E.; and Williams, T.J. (1973). Factors influencing survival in stage I ovarian cancer. *Am J Obstet Gynecol* **116:**222–228.

102. Webb, M.J.; Malkasian, G.D.; and Jorgensen, E.O. (1974). Factors influencing ovarian cancer survival after chemotherapy. *Obstet Gynecol* **44:**564–570.

103. Wharton, J.T. (1976). Principles of surgical and irradiation treatment for carcinoma of the ovary. In *Gynecologic Oncology*, Rutledge, F.N.; Boronow, R.C.: and Wharton, J.T., (Eds.) Wiley, New York, pp. 177–182.

104. Wilson, W. L.; Bisel, H.F.; Cole, D.; Rochlin, D.; Ramirez, G.; and Madden, R. (1970). Polonged low-dosage administration of hexamethylmelamine (NC—13875). *Cancer* **25:**568–570.

105. Wiltshaw, E.; and Carr; B. (1974). Cis-Platinum (II) diamminedichloride: clinical experience of the Royal Marsden Hospital and Institute of Cancer Research, London. *Recent Results Cancer Res* **45:**178–182.

106. Wiltshaw, E.; and Kroner, T. (1976). Phase II study of Cis-Dichlorodiammine-platinum (II) (NSC—119875) in advanced adenocarcinoma of the ovary. *Cancer Treat Rep* **60:**55–60.

107. Young, R.C.; Chabner, B.A.: Hubbard, S.P.; Fisher, R.I.; Bender, R.A.; Anderson, T.; and DeVita, V.T. (1978). Advanced ovarian adenocarcinoma: Melphalan (PAM) vs. combination chemotherapy (Hexa-CAF). *Proc Am Soc Clin Oncol* **346.**

108. Young, R.C.: Canellos, G.P.; Chabner, B.A.: Schein, P.S.; Hubbard, S.P.; and DeVita, V.T. (1974). Chemotherapy of advanced ovarian carcinoma: a prospective randomized comparison of phenyl-alanine mustart and high dose cyclophosphamide. *Gynecol Oncol* **2:**489–497.

109. Young, R.C. (1975). Chemotherapy of ovarian cancer: past and present. *Semin Oncol* **2:**267–276.

Immediate Versus Delayed Lymph-Node Dissection in Stage I Melanoma of the Limbs

U. Veronesi

Istituto Nazionale dei Tumori and WHO Collaborating Centres for Evaluation of Methods of
Diagnosis and Treatment of Melanoma,
Milan, Italy*

TREATMENT OF HUMAN MALIGNANT MELANOMA is still a subject of controversy, with many questions still awaiting a convincing answer. Among them are the extent of surgical removal of the skin surrounding the tumor, the removal of underlying fascia, the technique of surgical dissection of lymph nodes (if in continuity or in discontinuity with the primary), the timing of lymph-node dissection, whether prophylactic or therapeutic, the role of adjuvant chemotherapy, the place of immunotherapy, the possibilities of regional perfusion with chemotherapeutic agents, and of hyperthermia.

From the surgical point of view the most discussed question is whether or not to perform an elective lymph-node dissection in cases with clinically uninvolved regional lymph nodes. Such a procedure is considered necessary in most cases by some authors, whereas others are convinced that the prognosis is no worse if dissection is performed only after the appearance of metastases at the regional nodes. To reach an answer to this question, a controlled therapeutic trial was conducted from September 1967 to January 1974 by the WHO International Melanoma Group, involving 17 cancer institutions in 12 countries. The results of this multicenter international trial, which consisted of 553 cases of malignant melanoma of the limbs, classified as $T_{1-2-3}N_0M_0$ according to the Tumor-Node-Metastasis (TNM) classification then in force, were reported in 1977.[†]

---

* Institutes participating in the trial consisted of the following: Cancer Research Centre of the USSR Academy of Medical Sciences, Moscow, USSR; Fondazione Pascale, Naples, Italy; Herzen State Oncological Institute, Moscow, USSR; Het Nederlands Kankerinstituut, Amsterdam, Netherlands; Hospital A.C. Camargo, São Paolo, Brazil; Instituto Nacional de Enfermedades Neoplásticas, Lima, Peru; Institut Gustave Roussy, Villejuif, France; Institut Jules Bordet, Brussels, Belgium; Istituto Nazionale Tumori, Milan, Italy; Norwegian Radium Hospital, Oslo, Norway; Oncological Research Institute, Sofia, Bulgaria; Oncological Institute, Cracow, Poland; Oncological Institute, Gliwice, Poland; Oncological Institute, Warsaw, Poland; Oncological Institute, Brno, Czechoslovakia; Petrov Research Institute of Oncology, Leningrad, USSR; and State Institute of Oncology, Budapest, Hungary.

† U. Veronesi et al. (1977). Inefficacy of immediate node dissection in stage I melanoma of the limbs. *N Engl Med,* **297**:627–30.

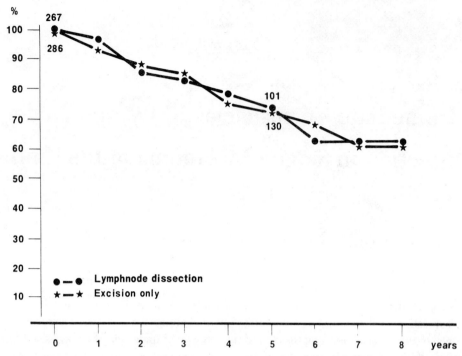

Fig. 1. Survival of 553 cases of malignant melanoma $T_{1-3}N_0M_0$ of the extremities, according to type of treatment.

Lower-limb and upper-limb melanomas, classified as $T_{1-2-3}N_0M_0$ only, not more than 5 cm in largest dimension and without fixation to the fascia, were included in the trial. Cases with satellite nodules were included when the nodules were within an area that did not exceed 5 cm and comprised that of the primary melanoma. Only cases that had never been treated or in which the previous treatment consisted in excisional biopsy of the primary tumor less than four weeks before admission to the trial were included.

Patients were assigned to one or the other group (excision only or excision combined with immediate regional lymph-node dissection) at random. To prevent a bias from differences in operating technique, cases were randomized within each collaborating center. Patients in whom a previous biopsy of primary melanoma had been performed were separately randomized.

Only cases with adequate histologic diagnosis were included in the trial. In all cases, the original diagnosis made by a local pathologist was reviewed by a panel of five pathologists, including a pathologist designated by the WHO Reference Center on Skin Tumors. Out of the original 557 cases submitted, 4 were considered questionable or doubtful and were not accepted.

Of the 553 cases of malignant melanoma of the limbs classified as $T_{1-2-3}N_0M_0$, 490 were untreated, and 63 had undergone limited excision of the primary melanoma less than four weeks before definitive treatment; 103 patients were male, and 450 female.

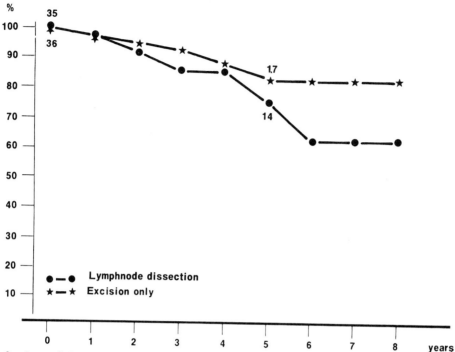

Fig. 2. Survival of 71 cases of malignant melanoma of the extremities $T_{1-3}N_0M_0$, Clark's level III, according to type of treatment.

Excision with immediate lymph-node dissection was performed in 267 patients, and excision of the primary melanoma only in 286.

The graph of Figure 1 shows no difference in survival within the two groups. The patients who underwent immediate node dissection and those subjected to regional lymph-node dissection when node dissection became clinically evident were well balanced according to previous biopsy, sex and age, site of origin, and histology. No difference was found in the survival rate obtained with elective node dissection as compared to that obtained with the delayed one, even when considering each subgroup of cases. In particular, the survival observed after the two types of treatment was not different for level III and IV cases (Figs. 2 and 3). The comparative incidence of regional lymph-node metastases, both occult at the time of elective node dissection and developed after excision only of the primary melanoma, is superimposable (19.7 and 24.2%, respectively, $P = 0.27$). The analysis was done only on cases treated before December 1971 in order to have a sufficient follow-up period and to consider the figures for patients subjected to excision only practically as final. The difference in five-year survival observed in N_0+ patients (36.8%) and in patients who developed regional node metastases (30.2%) was not statistically significant when evaluated from the time of treatment of the primary melanoma ($P = 0.57$).

It was concluded that elective node dissection does not improve the prognosis of MM of the limbs. Since the percentage of positive nodes ranges from 20 to 25%, the wait-and-see

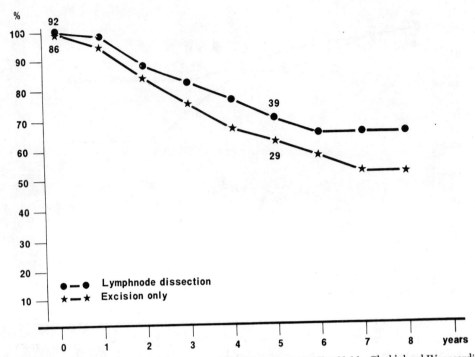

Fig. 3. Survival of 178 cases of malignant melanoma of the extremities $T_{1-3}N_0M_0$, Clark's level IV, according to type of treatment.

policy avoids unnecessary postoperative complications in three-fourths of the patients, for whom prophylactic dissection would result in the negative histologic finding of regional nodes. It was, however, stressed that delayed node dissection is advisable as long as the patients can be examined quarterly.

Efficacy of Elective Regional Lymph-Node Dissection in Primary (Stage I) Malignant Melanoma

F. J. Lejeune

Department of Surgery
Institut Jules Bordet
Bruxelles, Belgium

INTRODUCTION

THE EFFICACY OF ELECTIVE regional lymph-node dissection in primary (stage I) malignant melanoma is the center of a current controversy. This is not the case for stage IIb, when regional lymph nodes are found to be invaded: it is widely accepted that a radical lymph-node dissection should be performed with therapeutical intent. However, this procedure will only cure about 30% of cases. In contrast, for stage I, when regional lymph nodes do not clinically appear to be involved, node dissection should be considered either as a adjunctive treatment to wide excision of the primary or as a staging procedure. Here is the crucial problem in the controversy: it seems clear to us that the latter started with a misunderstanding. There are indeed two grounds for the controversy: therapeutical efficacy vs staging procedure. In most debates on the problem there has been an obvious confusion with the two different aspects. We strongly feel that the two aspects should be discussed separately. Therefore we shall try to reply to two different questions: Does elective regional lymph node dissection provide (1) a therapeutical benefit and (2) essential information on regional lymph nodes for the staging of the disease?

ELECTIVE LYMPH NODE DISSECTION AS A TREATMENT

In the year 1960, the thesis on malignant melanoma was that it is a rapidly aggressive tumor justifying any form of surgical treatment. Some authors indeed recommended major amputations for melanoma of the limbs.[7,18] As regional lymph nodes can become metastatic, it was believed that immediate dissection with the primary would provide a better chance of cure. Most unselected series of stage I malignant melanoma showed around 25% of microscopical invasion of the clinically normal regional lymph nodes (N_{0+}).[6,7,8,10,13,17,20,25]

What is the evidence for therapeutical efficacy?

Only retrospective or prospective, but not randomized, studies brought about a therapeutic benefit.

Retrospective or prospective but not randomized studies

Nine studies (Table I) on unselected N_0 (stage I, with clinically uninvolved lymph nodes) were published between 1958 and 1976.

In 1958, Lane et al.[12] claimed a longer survival (60%) in patients with nonpalpable lymph nodes (N_0) submitted to large excision plus elective lymph-node dissection, as compared (10%) with patients submitted to the same treatment, but presenting with clinically involved lymph nodes (N_1). Lehman et al.[13] found no difference in treating N_0 patients either with wide excision or with excision and elective lymph-node dissection. However, they found a much higher survival rate (71%) in N_{0-} patients (microscopically free of metastases) as

TABLE I
Five-Year Survival Rate Percentage in Unselected N_0 (Stage I) Cases

Year	Authors	Large excision only	Large excision + elective lymph-node dissection	Therapeutic lymph-node dissection
1958	Lane et al.[12]	—	60	10
1964	Fortner et al.[7]	—	N_{0-}:78.3	—
			N_{0+}:22.7	
1965	Mundth et al.[17]	—	N_{0-}:77	
			N_{0+}:59	22
1966	Lehman et al.[13]	50	46	
			N_{0-}:71	
			N_{0+}:17	14
1967	Conley[a 6]	62	76	
			N_{0+}:25	14.6
1970	Goldsmith et al.[8]	68	78	
			N_{0+}:48	—
1971	Polk et al.[21] (survey)	70	N_{0+}:39	29
1974	Gumport and Harris[10]	—	N_{0+}:30	10
1976	Southwick[25]	—	N_{0-}:47	
			N_{0+}:30	18

[a] Head and neck melanoma only.

compared with N_{0+} patients (microscopically invaded regional lymph nodes), where they have had five-year survival rate of 17%. Such a difference between N_{0-} and N_{0+} patients was a confirmation of the earlier findings by Fortner et al. in 1964.[7] Further demonstration of the strong selective effect of nodal histological staging in N_0 patients was brought out by the works of Mundth et al.,[17] Conley,[6] Goldsmith et al.,[8] and Southwick.[25]

When the N_{0-} patients were compared to the N_0 patients, a 21% higher survival[13] was found in the first group. The same *a posteriori* comparison could be made between N_{0+} patients and N_1 patients treated by therapeutical lymph-node dissection. All six studies showed an improvement in favor of elective lymph-node dissection: 3%, 10%, 10%, 12%, 20%, and 37%, respectively.

Despite this trend in favor of elective lymph-node dissection, the conclusions of such retrospective studies should be taken with great caution. The comparison was made between *a posteriori* highly selected patients—on clinical and histological criteria—and the controls, which were historical. Therefore, the therapeutic benefit of elective lymph-node dissection was not definitively proved, as no criteria for selecting high-risk patients had been used in these studies (Table 1).

In contrast, the pionneering work if Mehnert et al.[16] in 1965 provided a method for discerning primary melanoma with poor survival. It was already based on histological in-filtration of the skin. Since then, the works of Clark[4] and Breslow[2] provided the melano-mologists with highly valuable methods for histological grading of primary malignant melanoma. Patients preselected as having a poor prognosis, according to these methods, and who were submitted to elective lymph-node dissection had a longer survival than those submitted to wide excision only. However, these studies were not randomized; therefore, the conclusion can only be considered as trends in favor of elective lymph-node dissec-tion.

Table II displays the survival rates obtained in three different grades, adapted from Mehnert's classification to Clark's. From this work it seems that only grades III and IV benefited from elective lymph-node dissection, while grade V was not at all improved by removal of lymph nodes. Ten years later, the study by Wanebo et al.[29] using the Clark classification confirmed these earlier findings. In addition, when the groups of cases with elective lymph-node dissection were broken down into N_{0-} and N_{0+}, it was apparent that N_{0+} at grade IV were no longer improved (Table II).

In contrast to the Clark method, which uses histological landmarks, Breslow's grading is based on the assessment of actual melanoma thickness where thresholds can build up: both Breslow's[2,3] and Hansen et al's.[11] data demonstrated that patients with melanoma of less than 1.5 mm would not benefit from elective lymph-node dissection. In contrast, with a melanoma reaching 1.5 mm in thickness, the patient submitted to node dissection will experience a 30% increase in survival rate (from 31% to 64% and from 53% to 82%, re-spectively). Despite the fact that these two works were promising for selecting patients to benefit from dissection, they were not randomized and therefore need to be confirmed by controlled studies.

Randomized Studies

Two recent prospective and randomized trials provided a negative answer. In the trial

TABLE II
Selection by Microstaging: Five-Year Survival Percentage

Year	Authors	Microstaging	Large excision only	Large excision + lymph-node dissection
1965	Mehnert et al.[16]	III[a]	77.2	100
		IV	25	75
		V	25	0
1974	Hansen and McCarten[11]	<1.5 mm[b,c]	100	90
		≥1.5 mm	53	82
1975	Breslow[3]	<.76 mm[b]	100	100
		>1.5 mm	31	64
1975	Wanebo et al.[29]	II[d]	100	100
				N_{0-}:100[e]
				N_{0+}:100
		III	67	93
				N_{0-}: 91
				N_{0+}:100
		IV	57	68
				N_{0-}: 82
				N_{0+}: 27
		V	50	0
				N_{0-}: 0
				N_{0+}: 0

[a] Adapted to the Clark's classification.
[b] Tumor thickness by micrometer.
[c] Head and neck melanoma only.
[d] Clark's classification.
[e] N_0: lymph nodes not palpable: N_{0-}: and histologically negative; N_{0+}: and histologically positive.

conducted by the WHO Malignant Melanoma Group, no difference was found in survival[27] between the group with elective lymph-node dissection and the group with wide excision only. In the same way, preliminary results of a trial from the Mayo Clinic[24] show equal survival when immediate or delayed elective lymph-node dissection were performed or when wide local excision was the only treatment.

It should be pointed out, however, that the WHO trial[27] was initiated in 1967, when no established histological grading was available. Therefore no selection of high-risk patients had been made: all patients presenting with any melanoma of the limbs were included in the study.

TABLE III
Selected Results from WHO Melanoma Trial No. 1 (Ref. 27)[a]

Criterion	Large excision only	Large excision + lymph-node dissection
Males	55.9	64.7
Maximum diameter		
11–20 mm	63	77.1
Upper limbs	45.3	54.7
Clark grade 4	58.3	70.1
Breslow >1.5 mm	69.7	78.5

[a] Five-year survival percentage.

267 patients underwent radical excision of the primary and repair with graft, 286 patients had, in addition to it, an elective radical regional lymph-node dissection. From the 101 survivors in the first group and the 130 in the second, it was concluded that no significant difference could be detected, as the curves were similar. However, some criticism arises when population sampling is looked at. First of all this trial only admitted patients with malignant melanoma of the limbs (83% of lower limbs). That is a preferential localisation in females, who predominated (81%). The large angle survival curves, so far obtained, might well hide a difference, which could be detected later in the following up of the patients.

Secondly, the Clark and/or Breslow grading was only done in 283 out of the 553 cases, which is less than half of the series. This is also a gap that might introduce a very dangerous bias in the analysis.

Notwithstanding this lack of information, which presumably is going to be solved in further analysis, some trends, in the published analysis, in favor of elective lymph-node dissection emerge (Table III). There is an apparent but not significant benefit of elective lymph-node dissection as compared to radical excision of the primary only, as there is around a 10% increase in the five-year survival rate (see also Ref. 9) in males, in the upper extremities, in tumors of 11–20 mm in diameter, in Clark grade 4 and in Breslow 1.6–4.5 mm in thickness.

It is interesting to point out that the benefit is precisely in categories of patients where the prognosis is severe: males and Clark and Breslow high-risk melanoma. In the latter, these results tend to confirm the earlier, nonrandomized studies that were referred to previously, that is, benefit from elective lymph-node dissection in Clark IV and Breslow thicker than 1.5 mm.

Therefore this trial,[27] together with the more recent report from the Mayo Clinic,[24] only shows that unselected patients with limb melanoma do not benefit from elective lymph-node dissection and there are quite a few arguments from the data in favor of a benefit in selected high-risk melanoma.

Therefore, the selection of poor-risk primary melanoma, according to histological grading, for performing elective lymph-node dissection looks justifiable in current or future randomized trials.

TABLE IV
Prognosis Factors in Stage I Melanoma (Five-Year Survival). a. Clinical Factors[a]

Sex	
Males:	42%
Females:	58%
Localization	
Head and neck:	52%
Arm:	60%
Leg:	58%
Trunk:	42%
Clinical type	
Lentigo malignant melanoma:	80%
Superficial spreading melanoma:	69%
Nodular melanoma:	53%

[a] Adapted from Refs. 15 and 29.

ELECTIVE LYMPH-NODE DISSECTION AS A STAGING PROCEDURE IN STAGE I MELANOMA

Some prognostic factors are usually recognized in primary (stage I) malignant melanoma (Table I). Females have an overall better prognosis than males.[8,9,10] Melanoma of the extremities appears less lethal than the central areas[8] (Table IV).

Within the clinical type, melanoma arising on Dubreuilh (DM) Hutchinson melanosis provide longer survival than superficial spreading melanoma (SSM), which allows in turn a better survival than nodular melanoma (NM). It is well accepted that the Clark[4] and Breslow[2] histological grading methods represent the best prognosis criteria (Table V). We would like to demonstrate that the histological status of regional lymph nodes is an additional valuable criteria.

Table V, adapted from unpublished data from the WHO trial No. 1, clearly indicates that patients found with clinically uninvolved but histologically invaded lymph nodes, experienced a much shorter survival time. Such poor-risk patients represented about 20% of all cases with stage I melanoma. If the Clark or Breslow histological grading is taken into account, one could detect a population with higher frequency of histologically involved lymph nodes. As it is shown in Table VI, patients with melanoma of grade III (compiled by Veronesi[28]) or with a thickness greater than 3.1 mm[29] will have occult lymph-node metastasis in nearly 50% of them. This means that elective lymph-node dissection will change the clinical stage from I to II for 50% of readily selected patients.

The argument presented in 1971[20,21] that elective lymph-node dissection harmed 34/1,000 and benefitted 30/1,000 patients no longer appears tenable.

First of all, the 33% morbidity can be lowered to less than 5% if one performs a radical lymph-node dissection with a technique avoiding a delay in wound healing and subsequent lymphoedema.[26] Secondly, the only hope for improving the poor results of malignant melanoma treatment is in adjuvant treatments after surgery. Such treatments, involving either prophylactic chemotherapy or immunotherapy or both, are currently being studied,

TABLE V
Prognosis Factors in Stage I Melanoma (Five-Year Survival). b. Histological Factors[a]

Histological grading

Clark		Breslow	
II	72.2%	0–0.5	100%
III	46.5%	0.6–1.0	100%
IV	31.6%	1.1–1.5	89%
V	12%	1.6–2	82%
		2.1–3.0	58%
		>3.1	55%

Histological status of regional lymph nodes[b]

	Frequency	Five-Year Survival Percentage
N_{0-}	80.3%	69%
N_{0+}	19.7%	39%

[a] Adapted from Refs. 15 and 29.
[b] From WHO Ct No. 1 Primary Melanoma.

but the results are still too preliminary.[14] Performing elective lymph-node dissection would allow early detection[14] of stage II (locoregional spreading) melanoma patients, who therefore might benefit from an early adjuvant treatment. This attitude is being followed in the EORTC trial,[14] for melanoma of the limbs, and is confirmed by others.[1,9,22]

Finally the statement that removing regional lymph nodes might impair the regional antitumour immunity is supported neither by experimental facts nor by clinical trials.[27]

Therefore, it still seems justifiable to perform elective lymph-node dissection for advanced Clark-Breslow lesions,[9] specially if an early adjuvant treatment is planned for, in properly randomized trials.

TABLE VI
Incidence of N_{0+} According to Levels of Invasion

Clark[a]	N_{0+}	Breslow[b]	N_{0+}
II	5–25%	0–0.5	0%
		0.6–1.0	9%
III	4.3–26.6%	1.1–1.5	5%
		1.6–2.0	8%
IV	12.8–58.6%	2.1–3.0	22%
		>3.1	39%
V	40.9–75%		

[a] Compiled by Veronesi.[28]
[b] From Wanebo.[29]

SUMMARY

The controversy on elective lymph-node dissection appears to be based on two different aspects: elective lymph-node dissection(1) as a treatment and (2) as a staging procedure. It seems that this surgical technique has no overall therapeutic efficiency. However, it might improve survival in Clark III, IV, and V levels and in melanoma with more than a 1.5-mm thickness. The immediate regional lymph-node dissection, for melanoma of the limbs, provides valuable information about the histological status of the lymph nodes. In histologically selected patients, this surgical procedure can change the clinical stage from I (primary) in II (regional spread). The early detection of poor-risk patients might therefore allow an earlier adjuvant treatment, theoretically with better chance of efficacy. This attitude appears today only justified in randomized prospective trials.

ACKNOWLEDGMENT

The author wishes to thank Drs. J. Colon and co-workers, E. Macher, H. Schraffordt Koops, E. van Slooten, U. Veronesi and members of EORTC and WHO Melanoma Groups for the many valuable discussions on this subject.

REFERENCES

1. Balch, C. (1978). Discussion. In *Melanoma Conference NIH* Louie, A.; Davis, H.; and Jacobs, E. (Eds.). p. 8.
2. Breslow, A. (1970). Thickness, cross-sectional areas and depth of invasion in the prognosis of cutaneous melanoma. *Ann Surg* 172:902–908.
3. Breslow, A. (1975). Quoted by W. S. McCune in discussion of paper by Wanebo *et al.* (see Ref. 20).
4. Clark, W. H.; From, L.; Bernardino, E. A.; and Mihn, M. C. (1969). The histogenesia and biologic behaviour of primary human malignant melanomas of the skin. *Cancer Res* 29:705–727.
5. Cochran, A. J. (1969). Malignant melanoma: review of 10 years' experience in Glasgow, Scotland. *Cancer* 23:1190–1199.
6. Conley, J. (1967). Melanoma of the head and neck. In *Proceedings of the International Workshop on Cancer of the Head and Neck,* Butterworths, London, pp. 106–113.
7. Fortner, J. G.; Booher, R. J.; and Pack, G. T. (1964). Results of groin dissection for malignant melanoma in 220 patients. *Surgery* 55:485–494.
8. Goldsmith, H. S.; Shaw, J. P.; and Kin, D. H. (1970). Prognostic significance of lymph node dissection in the treatment of malignant melanoma. *Cancer* 26:606–609.
9. Goldsmith, H. S. (1978). The increasing controversy of immediate lymph node dissection in melanoma (submitted for publication).
10. Gumport, S. L.; and Harris, M. N. (1974). Results of regional lymph node dissection for melanoma. *Ann Surg* 179:105–108.
11. Hansen, M. G.; and McCarten, A. B. (1974). Tumor thickness and lymphocytic infiltration in malignant melanoma of the head and neck. *Am J Surg* 128:557–561.
12. Lane, N.; Lattes, B.; and Malm, J. (1958). Clinicopathological correlation in a series of 117 malignant melanomas of the skin of adults. *Cancer* 11:1025–1043.
13. Lehman, J. A. (1966). Clinical study of forty-nine patients with malignant melanoma. *Cancer* 19:611–619.
14. Lejeune, F. J.; and DeWasch, G. (1978). Malignant melanoma. In: *Radomized Trials in Cancer: A Critical Review by Sites.* Staquet, M. (Ed.). Raven Press, New York, pp. 339–357.

15. Mastrangelo, M. J.; Clark, W. H.; Bellet, R. E.; and Berd, D. (1978). Cutaneous malignant melanoma: diagnosis, prognosis and conventional radical therapy. In *Immunotherapy of Cancer: Present Status in Man.* Terry; and Windhorst (Eds.). Raven Press, New York, pp. 1–17.

16. Mehnert, J. H.; and Heard, J. L. (1965). Staging of malignant melanomas by depth of invasion. A proposed index to prognosis. *Am J Surg* **110**:168–176.

17. Mundth, E. D.; Guralnick,E. A.; and Raker, J. W . (1965). Malignant melanoma. A clinical study of 425 cases. *Ann Surg* **162**:15–28.

18. Pack, G. T.; and Ariel, I. M. (1957). Treatment of malignant melanoma by adequate (radical) surgical resection and radical amputation when indicated. In *Current Surgical Management.* Mulholland, Ellison, and Freison (Eds. Saunders, Philadelphia, pp. 438–446.

19. Pack, G. T. (1959). End results in the treatment of malignant melanoma. *Surgery* **46**:447–460.

20. Polk, H. J., Jr.; and Linn, B. S. (1971). Selective regional lymphadenectomy for melanoma: a mathematical aid to clinical judgment. *Ann Surg* **174**:402–413.

21. Polk, H. C., Jr. (1976). Adjunctive treatment for malignant melanoma. In: Controversy in Surgery. Varco, R. L.; and Delaney, J. P. (Eds.). Saunders, Philadelphia, pp. 211–221.

22. Raker, J. (1977). Discussion. In *Melanoma Conference NIH* Ed. Louie, A.; Davis, H.; and Jacobs, E. (Eds.). p. 7.

23. Sacre, R.; and Lejeune, F. J. (1978). Pattern of metastasis distribution in 173 melanoma patients as detected during the follow-up after treatment for stage I or II melanoma. In *Proceedings of the Fourth International Symposium Malignant Melanoma* (in press).

24. Sim, F. H.; Ivins, J. C.; and Taylor, W. P. (1977). A prospective randomized study of the efficacy of routine prophylactic lympho-adenectomy in the management of malignant melanoma: preliminary results. In: *13th Annual Meeting Society of Surgical Oncology,* pp. 159–160.

25. Southwick, H. W.; Slaughter, D. P.; Hinkamp, J. F.; and Johnson, F. E. (1962). The role of regional node dissection in the treatment of malignant melanoma. *Arch Surg* **85**:79–84.

26. Vander Ploeg, E.; and Schraffordt Koops, H. (1972). A modified technique of groin dissection. *Arch Chir Neerl* **24**:31–36.

27. Veronesi, U. et al. (1977). Inefficacy of immediate node dissection in stage I melanoma of the limbs. *N Engl J Med* **297**:627–630.

28. Veronesi, U.; Cascinelli, N.; Orefice, S.; and Vaglini, M. M. (1977). Surgical treatment of malignant melanoma of the skin. In: *Symposium on Recent Advances in the Diagnosis and Treatment of Malignant Melanoma.* Svejda, J. (Ed.), pp. 28–38.

29. Wanebo, H. J.; Fortner, J. G.; Woodruff, J.; MacLean B.; and Binkowski, E. (1975). Selection of the optimum surgical treatment of stage I melanoma by depth of microinvasion: use of the combined microstage technique (Clark-Breslow). *Ann Surg* **182**:302–315.

Levamisole Immunotherapy:
Basis and Clinical Trials in Cancer Patients

F. Martin

Laboratoire d'Immunologie
CNRS era 628, Faculté de Médecine,
Dijon, France

LEVAMISOLE [L-2,3,5,6-tetrahydro-6-phenylimidazo-(2-1b)-thiazole, hydrochloride] is a pure chemical, first used as an antihelminthic drug. An effect on immune response has been claimed by Renoux & Renoux,[8] who reported that levamisole enhanced immunization of mice against *Brucella abortus*. Since this first observation, levamisole has been considered to be a new immunostimulatory compound and has been used in a variety of clinical situations: bacterial and viral chronic infections, rheumatic diseases, and cancer.

IMMUNOLOGICAL BASIS OF LEVAMISOLE IMMUNOTHERAPY

It is still difficult to attribute a definite immunological effect to levamisole. Various reports (included or quoted by Chirigos[3]) have suggested that levamisole could have an enhancing effect on B lymphocytes (by increasing antibody production and the number of plaque-forming cells), on T lymphocytes (by increasing lymphocyte mitogen response, lymphokine production, graft versus host reaction, and the delayed hypersensitivity reaction) or on macrophages (by modifying chemotaxis and phagocytosis). However, the data are often conflicting, poorly documented, or establish only borderline effects.

Levamisole has also been described as an antianergic agent, restoring normal immune functions in immunosuppressed situations (e.g., advanced tumors or chronic infections). Tripodi et al.[14] have found that levamisole could render positive a negative delayed hypersensitivity reaction to dinitrochlorobenzene in cancer patients; however, it had no definite effect on tuberculin hypersensitivity. A restoration of delayed hypersensitivity reactions in cancer patients following levamisole treatment was also reported by Verhaegen et al.,[15]

Rojas et al.,[10] and Lewinski et al.[5] This was not confirmed by Lichtenfeld, Wiernik, and Shortridge[6] or by Hirshaut et al.[4]

EXPERIMENTAL BASIS OF LEVAMISOLE CANCER IMMUNOTHERAPY

The effect of levamisole on experimental tumors has recently been reviewed by Amery, Rojas, and Chirigos (personal communication). The results of this study show that: a) levamisole has a variable effect on tumor growth, either favorable, neutral, or unfavorable (tumor enhancement); b) the effect of levamisole on tumor growth may be dose-dependent, since the best results were obtained with doses of 2.5 or 5 mg/kg; c) it may be more effective in the treatment of slow-growing malignancies; d) levamisole may be more efficient in preventing metastasis than in treating primary tumors; and e) levamisole may be of more use when given as adjuvant treatment, complementing treatment by surgery or radiotherapy. This study concludes that levamisole is effective, at least when used under optimal conditions. However, the conclusion is made on the basis of an analysis of published reports and does not take into consideration the well-known fact that negative or unfavorable results are less often submitted and accepted for publication than are more optimistic data. In an experiment by the author, levamisole, 2.5 mg/kg, was found to have no effect on the recurrence rate or on the occurrence of lung metastasis when given as an adjuvant to surgical excision of a slow-growing intestinal carcinoma in rat (Martin and Martin, unpublished results).

CLINICAL DATA: ADMINISTRATION SCHEDULES

In clinical trials, levamisole was given orally, at a daily dose of 150 mg/kg, on either two consecutive days, weekly, or on three consecutive days every other week. This schedule is not the result of a rational, phase I trial but represents the transposition to cancer immunotherapy of schedules used for the treatment of infectious or rheumatic diseases.

CLINICAL DATA: SIDE EFFECTS AND TOXICITY

Side effects occur frequently in levamisole-treated patients: nausea, vomiting, diarrhaea, agitation, insomnia, urticarial skin rash and flu-like illness with fever are seen. These effects were severe enough to stop therapy in 15 of 69 patients (Parkinson et al.[7]) and in 29 of 174 patients (Teerenhovi et al.[13]) in two series of trials in which levamisole was given for cancer immunotherapy. However, these side effects disappeared rapidly when levamisole therapy was stopped.

A more serious, potentially mortal complication of levamisole treatment is agranulocytosis or severe granulopenia. Its outbreak is often sudden, with clinical symptoms of septicemia. Levamisole-dependent leucoagglutinins have been found in the serum of such patients. Clinical and hematological improvement was usually rapid when levamisole therapy was stopped immediately and definitively and the septicaemia treated with broad-spectrum antibiotics, but lethal evolutions have been reported. Levamisole-induced agranulocytosis has been claimed to be more frequent in patients treated for rheumatic diseases; however, since the first case was published (Parkinson et al.[7]), it has been reported with considerable frequency (3 of 14 and 17 of 174 patients) in connection with cancer immunotherapy (Retsas et al.;[9] Teerenhovi et al.[13]).

EFFICACY OF CANCER IMMUNOTHERAPY WITH LEVAMISOLE

We are aware of the results of three clinical trials of levamisole in cancer immuno-therapy.

A. Breast Cancer (Rojas et al.[11])

Forty-eight patients with breast cancer stage III (UICC classification) were treated primarily by radiation therapy (cobalt source). After completion of the therapy, patients were assigned alternately to either a control group, which received no further treatment, or to a levamisole-treated group, which received 150 mg levamisole orally, three consecutive days every other week. The two groups were comparable with regard to age, menopausal status, and parity. The median disease-free interval was 8.9 months for the control group and 22.5 months for the treated group ($p = 0.01$). The median survival times were 22 months for the control group and 41.5 months for the treated group ($p = 0.05$). These results could suggest that levamisole is effective as an adjuvant to radiotherapy for treatment of breast cancer. However, it must be emphasized that the control and levamisole-treated groups were not allocated by randomization and that five patients, four of whom were in the levamisole-treated group, were lost for evaluation. Statistical bias could thus alter the significance of the results.

B. Lung Cancer (Amery[1,2])

At its last available report, this study included 148 patients who had entered the trial at least one year before evaluation. The patients were selected for presence of surgically resectable and histologically confirmed primary bronchogenic carcinoma. They were assigned randomly to one of two double-blind treatment groups, receiving either levamisole or a placebo. The drug was given orally at 150 mg daily for three consecutive days every two weeks. Statistical analysis of the total population showed only a slight trend favoring levamisole: actuarial curves for disease mortality and suspected recurrences differed significantly ($p = 0.05$) for a short period only, 18 to 21 months after surgery. The difference between both groups was considerably increased when only the patients who had a preoperative body weight of 70 kg or less were considered. This result was attributed to an underdosing of the patients who weighed more than 70 kg. However, this interpretation, and even the legitimacy of an a posteriori stratification, are fully questionable.

C. Malignant Melanoma (Spitler et al.[12])

At its last report, this study included 132 patients with primary or recurrent malignant melanoma with a poor prognosis. Patients were assigned to one of six groups on the basis of their clinical and pathological status, then randomized between levamisole- and placebo-treated groups. The drug was given double-blind on three consecutive days every two weeks (150 mg levamisole per day). Preliminary results of this trial showed no significant difference between actuarial curves for first recurrence, first visceral recurrence (metastasis), or survival.

CONCLUSIONS

At the present time, the use of levamisole in the routine treatment of cancer can be supported neither by clear-cut biological data that would establish its effect on the immune system, nor by convincing experimental results, nor by entirely reliable clinical trials. Two of the three available clinical trials suggest a favorable effect, but they are unfortunately obscured by methodological bias. Furthermore, the relatively high incidence of undesirable side-effects, including potentially mortal agranulocytosis, does not lend support to the early reputation of levamisole as a well-tolerated drug. From now on, levamisole should be proscribed as a routine treatment for cancer.

On the other hand, the noneffectiveness of levamisole in the treatment of human cancer has not been proven; levamisole should therefore be tested along with nonproven therapeutics, in well-conducted clinical trials in situations comparable to "optimal" experimental conditions (adjuvant therapy of slow-growing cancer). A number of new trials, now in progress, will probably resolve the question of the clinical usefulness of levamisole in cancer immunotherapy.

REFERENCES

1. Amery, W. (1976). Double-blind levamisole trial in resectable lung cancer. *Ann NY Acad Sci*, 277:260–68.

2. Amery, W. (1978). A placebo-controlled levamisole study in resectable lung cancer. In *Immunotherapy of Cancer: Present Status of Trials in Man*, W. D. Terry and D. Windhorst (eds.), Raven Press, New York, 191–201.

3. Chirigos, M. A., ed. (1977). *Control of Neoplasia by Modulation of the Immune System*, Raven Press, New York.

4. Hirshaut, Y.; Pinsky, C. M.; Krown, S. E.; Wanebo, H.; and Oettgen, H. F. (1977). Phase I evaluation of immune effects of levamisole. In *Control of Neoplasia by Modulation of the Immune System*. Chirigos M. A. (ed.), Raven Press, New York.

5. Lewinski, U. H.; Mavligit, G. M.; Gutterman, J. U.; and Hersh E. M. (1977): Administration of a single dose of levamisole to carcinoma patients: *in vivo* and *in vitro* enhancement of cellular immune response. In *Control of Neoplasia by Modulation of the Immune System*. M. A. Chirigos (ed.), Raven Press, New York.

6. Lechtenfeld, J. L.; Wiernik, P. H.; and Shortridge, D. G. (1977) Phase I trial of levamisole in patients with nonresectable bronchogenic carcinoma. In *Control of Neoplasia by Modulation of the Immune System*. M. A. Chirirgos (ed.), Raven Press, New York.

7. Parkinson, D. R.; Jerry, L. M.; Shibata, H. R.; Lewis, M. G.; Cano, P. O.; Capek, A.; Mansell, P. W.; and Marquis, G. (1977). Complications of cancer immunotherapy with levamisole. *Lancet*, II:1129–32.

8. Renoux, G., and Renoux, M. (1971). Effet immunostimulant d'un imidothiazole dans l'immunisation des souris contre l'infection par *Brucella abortus*. *C R Acad Sci* (Paris), 272:349–50.

9. Retsas, S.; Phillips, R. H.; Hanham, I. W. F.; and Newten, K. A. (1978). Agranulocytosis in breast cancer patients treated with levamisole. *Lancet*, **III**:324–25.

10. Rojas, A. F.; Mickiewicz, E.; Feierstein, J. N.; Glait, H.; and Olivari, A. J. (1976). Levamisole in advanced breast cancer. *Lancet*, **1**:211–15.

11. Rojas, A. F.; Feierstein, J. N.; Glait, H. M.; and Olivari, A. M. (1978). Levamisole action in breast cancer stage III. In *Immunotherapy of Cancer: Present Status of Trials in Man*, W. D. Terry and D. Windhorst (eds.), Raven Press, New York.

12. Spitler, L. E.; Sagebiel, R. W.; Glogau, R. G.; Wong, P. P.; Malm, T. M.; Chase, R. H.; and Gonzalez, R. L. (1978). A randomized double-blind trial of adjuvant therapy with levamisole *versus* placebo in patients with malignant melanoma. In *Immunotherapy of Cancer: Present Status of Trials in Man*. W. D. Terry and D. Windhorst (eds.), Raven Press, New York.

13. Teerenhovi, L.; Heinonen, E.; Gröhn, P.; Klefström, P.; Mehtonen, M.; and Tilikainen A. (1978). High frequence of agranulocytosis in breast cancer patients treated with levamisole. *Lancet*, **III**:151–52.

14. Tripodi, D.; Parks, L. C.; and Brugmans, J. (1978). Drug-induced restoration of cutaneous delayed hypersensitivity in anergic patients with cancer. *N Engl J Med*, **289**:354–57.

15. Verhaegen, H.; Verbruggen, F.; Verhaegen-Declercq, M. L.; and de Cree, J. (1974): Effets du lévamisole sur les réactions cutanées d'hypersensibilité retardée. *Nouv Presse Med*, **3**:2483–85.

CHAPTER 25

Clinical Trials of Levamisole in Humans

David P. Byar

Clinical and Diagnostic Trial Section
Biometry Branch
National Cancer Institute
Bethesda, Maryland U.S.A.

LEVAMISOLE WAS FIRST USED as an antihelminthic. Chemically it is an imidazothiazole derivative. About six years ago, it was learned that this drug may increase cellular immune reactivity in animals and man. Conflicting results have been obtained concerning the use of levamisole in tumor-bearing animals, but in several animals models prolonged disease remission, increased survival, and decreased incidence of metastases have been reported. In other experiments, no effects have been observed (see the chapter by F. Martin for details of preclinical studies).

So far as I am aware, this drug is the only chemically-defined substance which is currently in use as an immunologic agent for treating human cancers, although no doubt others are being studied. It is generally described as falling into the category of a nonspecific immunostimulant, and Symoens has referred to it as an anti-anergic chemotherapeutic agent.[1] The fact that it is chemically defined sets it apart from biologic substances such as BCG, C. Parvum, tumor vaccines, transfer factor, and a variety of other products, which have been used in attempts to influence the immunocompetence of patients with cancer. The drug may be given orally and it is generally considered to have minimal toxicity. In most of the studies I shall describe, bone-marrow toxicity has not been observed, and the principal problems seem to have been confined to nausea and vomiting, malaise, nervousness sometimes causing sleep disturbances, and shivering with or without fever. However, marrow suppression has occasionally been attributed to levamisole, but it was reversible when the drug was stopped.[2]

MALIGNANT MELANOMA

The rationale for the study by Spitler et al.[3] was based on their studies of Fortner's melanotic melanoma of the golden Syrian hamster. Levamisole did not affect the growth of the primary tumor, but it did impair growth of recurrent melanomas, curing one-third of the animals studied, a phenomena never noted in control animals. In addition, levamisole reduced the incidence of pulmonary metastasis by 50%. Accordingly they undertook a randomized clinical trial of patients with primary and recurrent melanoma of poor prognosis.

Patients were stratified into six groups on the basis of Clark's levels, results of lymph-node dissections, and the site of the tumor. Patients with level II, melanoma of the orbit, and those having had previous chemotherapy or radiotherapy were excluded. The study was conducted in a double-blind fashion using placebo tablets identical in appearance to 150 mg tablets of levamisole. Patients were instructed to take one tablet for three days in a row every two weeks for two years if there was no recurrence of their tumor. In the instance of recurrence, they were to continue taking the pill until they had been tumor free for two years or until death. Sixty-five patients were randomized to placebo and 67 to levamisole. Examination of the patient characteristics revealed a slight bias in favor of those assigned to levamisole with respect to sex (46% females for levamisole vs. 29% for placebo) and Clark's levels for the primary melanomas (62% levels IV–V for levamisole vs. 83% for placebo).

No significant difference was detected in duration of the disease-free interval, and the actuarial curves for the two treatment groups cross three times. Curves constructed for time-to-first-visceral recurrence and overall survival curves all have failed to reveal any significant differences. The authors concluded that to date their study had revealed no difference between levamisole at the dose studied and placebo in treating patients with primary or recurrent malignant melanoma. There do not appear to be any flaws in the design or execution of this study so far as one can judge from the written report.

STAGE III BREAST CANCER

Rojas et al.[4] have described a study of levamisole after radiotherapy for patients with stage III breast cancer. Radiotherapy delivered from a cobalt source consisted of 4,000 rad to both the chest wall and supraclavicular area and 3,000 rad to the posterior axillary field over a period of about two months. After completion of radiation therapy, patients were assigned alternately (rather than by randomization) either to a control group or to levamisole. The study was not double blinded and the control group received no further treatment until evidence of recurrent disease. Levamisole treatment consisted of 150 mg taken orally on three consecutive days every other week until evidence of progressive disease. The distributions of the patients in the two treatment groups according to age, age at menopause, and TNM classifications were similar.

A striking difference was noted in the length of disease-free intervals reported as significant at $p < .01$ by the generalized Wilcoxon test. The median disease-free interval for the levamisole group was 22.5 months vs. 8.9 months for the control group. Interestingly, a significantly higher frequency of lung metastasis was observed in the levamisole treated group (8/13 for levamisole vs. 5/23 for control).

The authors also report on a comparison of 33 levamisole-treated patients with 70 stage III historical controls. It is never clearly stated whether these 33 patients were different from the 20 patients in the controlled study, but it seems likely that this group of 33 patients included those 20 plus an additional 13 treated with levamisole after the completion of that study. The historical control patients were similar to the levamisole-treated patients with respect to age and menopausal age; however, the historical control group contained 40% of patients with T4 lesions, according to the TNM classification, versus only 24% in the levamisole-treated group. This fact could produce serious bias in comparing these two groups. Nevertheless the behavior of the historical control group was similar to that of the concurrent control group.

The authors reported that levamisole treatment was associated with an increase in the number of strong positive reactions to DNCD stimulation, but that not all patients increased in their reactions. Although no statistically significant results are claimed, the authors observed that patients whose reactions increased to strong positive showed the best clinical course, whereas those whose reactions remained negative had the worst evolution.

This study may be taken as providing encouraging evidence that levamisole treatment may be of benefit to patients with stage III breast cancer. However, it needs to be repeated at another center because of several methodological weaknesses. The first is that one is always suspicious of alternate assignment to treatment as opposed to randomization, because it gives the investigators the opportunity, whether consciously or unconsciously, to bias the assignment of treatment. Secondly, I have pointed out that the historical control group contained a larger proportion of T4 lesions, possibly invalidating those comparisons. Finally, this is a very small study and one would prefer to see it repeated with larger numbers and according to a more rigorous experimental design.

RESECTABLE LUNG CANCER

Amery has reported the results of a placebo-controlled study of levamisole in resectable lung cancer.[5] This was a double-blind study, and patients were randomized separately in each of three cooperative centers. The report I am describing is the fourth interim analysis and is based on 82 levamisole-treated patients and 96 placebo-treated patients who were operated on at least one year before the report was prepared. Levamisole was administered in 50 mg tablets given three times daily on the last three days before surgery and in similar three-day courses repeated every two weeks for two years thereafter, unless relapse occurred. No chemotherapeutic agents, corticosteroids, or radiotherapy were permitted unless a proven recurrence could be documented. The endpoints studied were the first suspicion of recurrence, the first proof of relapse, and death due to lung cancer.

When analyses for these three endpoints were performed using all patients in the study, a positive trend appeared to be present in favor of levamisole with respect to time till suspected recurrence or death due to carcinoma. However, when a separate analysis was performed on those patients weighing less than 70 kg, much more impressive results in favor of levamisole were detected with respect to remission duration and survival. Unfortunately the authors chose to analyze the survival data by computing Student's t-test at each three-month interval rather than using a composite test for comparing the whole survival curves, such as the log-rank test or the generalized Wilcoxon test. Nevertheless, the survival curves for those patients weighing less than 70 kg are sufficiently separated so that it is probable that significant results would have been obtained using these tests as well. They further commented, although the data are not presented in this report, that a positive trend was noted in each of the three centers, but no statistical analyses stratified by center, which might have allowed these positive trends to reinforce each other, are presented. They found no differences for their three major endpoints for patients weighing more than 70 kg. They commented that clinical results were better if the skin tests using PPD or DNCB were positive and for patients with larger tumors. They also found that levamisole was most effective in preventing blood-borne metastases as opposed to intrathoracic recurrences. The author feels that the results of this study indicate that a higher dose of levamisole should be used in future trials and suggests 2.5 mg per kg of body weight, or 100 mg per square meter of body-surface area.

This study raises interesting questions, which may possibly be answered in future studies. It is difficult to know how much belief to place in the study as reported. It is often possible to find significant differences in subsets of patients when overall there are no impressive differences. Whether this analysis qualifies as one of these instances is uncertain. I personally regard examining the data for patients under 70 kg as a sensible thing to do, since we know that the effect of most drugs depends on the dose and in this study a fixed dose was used, perhaps representing too small a dose in the heavier patients. However, I would have expected some effect in those weighting more than 70 kg, but the authors claim to have found none. An even more interesting question concerns the normal weight of these patients as opposed to their weight at the time they entered the trial. It is well known that even small lung cancers can lead to substantial reductions in body weight, perhaps by as much as 10 to 20% of normal body weight. If this was the case for those patients weighing less than 70 kg, we might wonder whether their tumors were more advanced and consequently they were more immunosuppressed, thus allowing them to benefit from the possible immunostimulant properties of levamisole. This would provide an alternate explanation to the notion that the heavier patients simply received too low a dose. Against this hypothesis, however, is the observation that most of the patients weighing less than 70 kg had positive skin tests to 100 micrograms of DNCB. No data were presented for those weighing more than 70 kg.

This study suggests that levamisole may be useful in the treatment of patients with resectable lung cancer, but most importantly it raises interesting questions which should be resolved in future studies.

STUDIES IN PROGRESS

I would like to describe briefly the progress to date in six on-going studies known to me only through personal communications or abstracts published just this month in the *Proceedings of the Joint Meeting of the American Association for Cancer Research and the American Society of Clinical Oncology*.

Smith et al.,[6] at UCLA, are carrying out a placebo-controlled double-blind trial of levamisole in patients with all stages of bladder cancer. Thus far they have randomized 31 patients with noninvasive bladder cancer and 23 patients with invasive disease. Levamisole has been administered by mouth at approximately 2.5 mg per kg of body weight on two sequential days each week. Patients have been followed from one month to more than two years. Thus far the investigators have observed no significant differences with respect to recurrence rates in either group of patients. The drug has been well tolerated with few side effects; however there were two instances of neutropenia. The protocol for this study calls for repeated skin testing with DNCB. They noted that approximately 80% of patients were negative prior to entry and that the percentage of positives increased at each three-month interval thereafter. Interestingly, they attributed the difference to the skin-testing procedure itself rather than to the therapy, an observation that should be kept in mind when interpreting the results of periodic skin testing in other protocols. It is obviously too early to draw any conclusions from this study, either negative or positive, concerning beneficial therapeutic effects of levamisole.

Pavlovsky et al.,[7] in Buenos Aires, Argentina, began a study in September, 1975, in which patients having achieved complete remission from acute lymphocytic leukemia were randomized to receive levamisole or not. It is not clear from their abstract whether this was a double-blind study, that is, whether a placebo was used. Levamisole was given in a dose of 100 mg per square meter of body surface area per day by mouth until relapse, as part of a maintenance therapy regime including 6-mercaptopurine and methotrexate with reinduction every three months with prednisone and vincristine. They have reported that 20 out of 86 patients receiving levamisole have relapsed compared to 36 out of 82 patients in the control group. The percentages in complete remission at one and two years for levamisole were 80% and 68% compared to 68% and 47% for those not receiving levamisole ($p < 0.05$). DNCB skin testing was also carried out in this study, and at 18 months 100% were positive in the levamisole group, versus 27% in the control group ($p < 0.005$). The authors believe that their results suggest that levamisole may prolong the duration of complete remission in acute lymphatic leukemia when used as an adjuvant to a chemotherapeutic maintenance regime.

Wanebo et al.,[8] at Sloan-Kettering in New York, have described a randomized trial comparing levamisole and placebo in patients with head and neck cancer after complete resection of the tumor. Randomization was stratified by site of the tumor, stage, and disease status at the time of surgery. Of 54 patients randomized, only 48 were evaluable. Among these, 9 had recurrent disease and 39 were treated for primary cancer. About 60% of those treated for primary cancer in both treatment groups received adjuvant radiotherapy. DNCB reactivity was similar for both patient groups. The authors claim that a significant reduction in recurrence rate was associated with levamisole treatment for patients with primary disease, but no differences have yet been observed for those treated for recurrent disease. At 12 months the estimated proportion free of disease was 34% in the placebo group versus 82% in the levamisole group, and the comparison of the recurrence distributions was significant at the $p < 0.025$. The estimated median recurrence time was nine months for the 21 patients receiving placebo and has not yet been reached for the 18 patients receiving levamisole. The authors feel that these preliminary results suggest that levamisole is of benefit as adjuvant treatment for patients with primary operable cancer of the head and neck. This is a very small study, but the results appear to be quite impressive. It will be interesting to see if the results hold up after more patients have been studied, and whether they can be confirmed in other centers.

Blumenschein et al.,[9] at M. D. Anderson Hospital in Houston, Texas, have described the results for 117 patients with metastatic breast cancer treated by FAC (5-fluorouracil, adriamycin, and cyclophosphamide), plus BCG administered by scarification, and levamisole, 100 mg per square meter by mouth on days 9, 10, 13, 14, 17, and 18 of every 21 days. Treatment results were compared with similar studies of patient populations with comparable prognostic factors treated with FAC alone, FAC-BCG, and FAC-levamisole. Randomization was not employed. The proportion of patients showing complete or partial response was about 70 to 75% in all four series, and a median duration of remission for FAC-BCG-levamisole (15 months) was similar to that for FAC-BCG or FAC-levamisole, but significantly longer than that for FAC alone (8.5 months). These results suggest that levamisole is active in prolonging the duration of remission in patients with advanced breast cancer when used as an adjuvant to three-agent chemotherapy. However, its effect was similar to that of BCG, and the two together offered no advantage over either one alone. Unfortunately, this study was not randomized, and no p-values are given in the abstract to help us evaluate the importance of an increase in the duration of remission from 8.5 to 15 months. Such a difference could easily result from the kinds of bias inherent in doing historically controlled studies. We may regard this study as showing some promise for levamisole, but the results should be confirmed in a randomized study.

Chang et al.,[10] at the NCI-Baltimore Cancer Research Center in Baltimore, Maryland, have compared results for 30 patients with acute nonlymphocytic leukemia treated by cytosine arabinoside and daunorubicin plus levamisole with those for 30 patients treated with the same two cyotoxic drugs without levamisole. It is not stated in the abstract that this was a randomized study. Levamisole was given in a dose of 45 mg per square meter twice a day for three days weekly from the second week of induction and continued until relapse or death. Fifty-three percent of patients in both groups achieved remission. Toxicity of levamisole was limited to transient nausea in occasional patients, but the drug was temporarily discontinued in eight patients with hepatic dysfunction. Eventually, it was decided that the hepatic dysfunction was unrelated to levamisole. At the time of writing their abstract, they stated that thus far levamisole appears to be of no additional benefit in this regimen, but that the chemotherapeutic regimen used achieved remission more rapidly and effectively than any they had previously studied. It is difficult to draw any conclusions concerning the role of levamisole in this study, first, because it may not have been randomized, and second, because the study is so small. In a study of this size it would be quite easy to miss important beneficial effects of levamisole.

Bedikian et al.,[11] of the M. D. Anderson Hospital in Houston, Texas, have studied levamisole in a randomized trial for patients with colorectal cancer. Four active agents were used sequentially (methotrexate, Baker's antifol, 5-fluorouracil, and methyl-CCNU). Levamisole was given at a dose of 150 mg per square meter by mouth on days 7, 8, 14, and 15 of each course of chemotherapy. Sixty previously untreated patients were studied. The authors note that levamisole did not increase survival or significantly influence the results of chemotherapy. Unfortunately, the numbers of patients studied are quite small and important differences could possibly have been missed. Even so, this study cannot be taken as providing encouraging evidence for a role of levamisole in the treatment of patients with colorectal cancer.

Although only sketchy details have been presented for the six studies reported in abstract, these results may be considered along with the three more detailed studies in evaluating the current status of levamisole. Of course, one should not interpret a study as negative if only a small number of patients have been studied and the results are preliminary, but in three of these six studies, significant differences in favor of levamisole already appear to have emerged. Thus, of the nine studies discussed in this presentation, five have indicated some benefit for levamisole: two in breast cancer, one in lung cancer, one in acute lymphocytic leukemia, and one in head and neck cancer. Overall these results suggest that levamisole certainly deserves further study, but it is too early to recommend its use in treating cancer patients except in a research setting. In addition, it seems wise that future research protocols should be both randomized and double blinded. Levamisole is an ideal drug for this kind of study, since the relative absence of toxic side effects makes it possible to blind the study with placebo tablets, as has been demonstrated in several of the studies reported here.

REFERENCES

1. Symoens, J. (1977). Levamisole: An anti-anergic chemotherapeutic agent. In *Control of Neoplasia by Modulation of the Immune System*, M. A. Chirigos (Ed), Raven Press, New York, 1–24.

2. Smith, R.B. Personal communication.

3. Spitler, L.E., et al. (1978). A randomized double-blind trial of adjuvant therapy with levamisole versus placebo in patients with malignant melanoma. In *Immunotherapy of Cancer: Present Status of Trials in Man*, W. D. Terry and D. Windhorst (Eds.), Raven Press, New York, 73–79.

4. Rojas, A.F., et al. (1978). Levamisole action in breast cancer stage III. In *Immunotherapy of Cancer: Present Status of Trials in Man*, W. D. Terry and D. Windhorst, (Eds.), Raven Press, New York, 635–45.

5. Amery, W.K. (1978). A placebo-controlled levamisole study in resectable lung cancer. In *Immunotherapy of Cancer: Present Status of Trials in Man*, W. D. Terry and D. Windhorst, (Eds.), Raven Press, New York, 191–99.

6. Smith, R.B. Personal communication.

7. Pavlovsky, S. (1978). Chemoimmunotherapy with levamisole in acute lymphocytic leukemia (Abstract 814). In *Proc Am Assoc Cancer Res*, **19**:March.

8. Wanebo, H.J., et al. (1978). Randomized trial of levamisole in patients with squamous cancer of head and neck (Abstract C-189). In *Proc Am Soc Clin Oncol*, **19**:March.

9. Blumenschein, G., et al. (1978). BCG plus levamisole immunotherapy with adriamycin combination chemotherapy of metastatic breast cancer. (Abstract C-393). In *Proc Am Soc Clin Oncol*, **19**:March.

10. Chang, P., et al. (1978). Levamisole, cytosine arabinoside, and daunorubicin induction therapy of adult acute nonlymphocytic leukemia. (Abstract C-254). In *Proc Am Soc Clin Oncol*, **19**:March.

11. Bedikian, A.Y., et al. (1978). Sequential chemoimmunotherapy of colorectal cancer: comparison of methotrexate, Baker's antifol, and levamisole. (Abstract C-446). In *Proc Am Soc Clin Oncol*, **19**:March.